Y0-BMD-204

**Bircher-Benner
Nutrition Plan
For Headache
and Migraine
Patients**

OTHER BIRCHER-BENNER HEALTH GUIDES:

Bircher-Benner Arthritis and Rheumatism Nutrition Plan
Bircher-Benner Nutrition Plan for Digestive Problems
Bircher-Benner Raw Food and Juices Nutrition Plan
Bircher-Benner Salt-Free Nutrition Plan

Bircher-Benner Nutrition Plan For Headache and Migraine Patients

A Comprehensive Guide With Suggestions for Diet Menus and Recipes

Translated by Timothy McManus

By the staff of the Bircher-Benner Clinic:

Medical/Dietetic Section:
D. Liechti-v. Brasch, M.D., P. F. Boesch, M.D., S. Grieder-Dopheide, M.D.

Physiological/Chemical Section:
Alfred Kunz-Bircher, Ph.D.

Menus and Recipes:
*Ruth Kunz-Bircher, M.D.
(head of the Bircher-Benner Clinic)*

Edited by *Ralph Bircher, M.D.*

NASH PUBLISHING • LOS ANGELES

Copyright © 1972 by Nash Publishing
originally published in German under the title
Bircher-Benner Handbuch, Kopfschmerzen und Migräne.
Copyright © 1959 by Bircher-Benner Verlag, Zürich, Bad Hamburg v.d.H.

All rights reserved. No part of this book
may be reproduced in any form or by any means
without permission in writing from the publisher.

Library of Congress Catalog Card Number: 77-186899
Standard Book Number: 8402-8031-9

Published simultaneously in the United States
and Canada by Nash Publishing Corporation, 9255 Sunset Boulevard,
Los Angeles, California 90069.

Printed in the United States of America.

First Printing.

About the Bircher-Benner Clinic

In the nineteenth century, Dr. M. Bircher-Benner wanted to establish a kind of clinic that had never existed before: a clinic that would take into account the whole man, both body and soul, not only the patient's disease; a clinic that would use an intelligent patient as a co-worker in a total therapeutic effort; a clinic that would use the total knowledge of modern medicine to support the "internal physician"–the autonomous healing forces and healing system of the body–and in every case make the healing effects of dietetic therapy and one's life-style the basis of a total health plan; a clinic that, in addition to eliminating immediate ailments, would bring about a new, tougher, more satisfying and creative health of body and soul for the patient.

The private clinic founded by Dr. Bircher-Benner in 1897 is still operated today for that purpose.

Contents

I. Headaches 1

II. Migraines 19

III. Menus 47

IV. Recipes 63

V. Exercises 153

I. Headaches

There are lucky people who have never in their lives experienced the torment and pain of a headache. Never have they felt their efficiency and vitality impaired by its onslaught. Unfortunately, these people are few in number. Contemporary man is well acquainted with the varied forms of headaches. He is familiar with them because of the internal and external strain placed upon him by his profession and social life and concerns; because of his poor habits that violate his own nature, turning night into day; because of his consumption of an excess of elaborately prepared, rich food and his rejection of whole grain and other healthy nourishment; and because of his unvarying dependence upon stimulants to help him overcome his fatigue, his aversion to his job, his restlessness, and his tension. In reaching for one of the many headache remedies, he loses sight of the real road to recovery in the forest of pain relievers.

Causes and Treatment

There are different varieties of headaches which are caused in different ways and are due to different kinds of illnesses. If one is to be genuinely and permanently helped, the person who is ill with a headache must be examined as a *whole:* the totality of his body and his personality.

Metabolic Overload

A feeling of heavy pressure over the brow and temples makes the eyes feel heavy and thinking laborious. It usually appears in the morning on waking, and often does not let up until the headache pill, which has unfortunately become a habit, takes effect. Without the pill, it increases during the day into genuine pain that torments and worries the sufferer and makes work requiring concentration impossible. In less severe cases, it lets up during breakfast or soon afterwards when work begins. In severe cases, it becomes unbearable and requires bed rest or medication.

This kind of headache is caused by metabolic overloading, poor circulation, the stimulant habit, and debased overrich food. A few illnesses, in which headaches are typical accompanying symptoms or warning signs, illustrate the close relationship between a headache and the body's general condition. Here, in all illnesses as well as in health, the whole person must not be forgotten in preoccupation with the symptoms of the disease. Every infirmity, including headaches, has its deeper roots in disturbances of the balance of body and mind. Treatments and life-style must take account of these deeper causes.

High Blood Pressure

As an example, take the so-called full-blooded person with high blood pressure, viscous (plethoric) blood, a florid complexion, and an angry streak in his personality, who gets riled up at the slightest irritation. It has become his habit to burden his bodily organs with deficient nourishment, an excess of fat and protein, white flour, sugar, nicotine, and other irritants. If he gets a headache, he should attend to it as a warning signal and regulate his life-style soon, otherwise he will have to count on an early old age and arteriosclerosis.

Arteriosclerosis

The old-age headache: Arteriosclerosis in aging people can also cause real headaches. The blood vessels which have been closed through rigidity and calcium deposits hamper the circulation of the blood to the head. The patient complains of vague discomforts, numbness, and mild to severe headaches from the nape of the neck to the forehead, which persist the entire day. In the morning, after the body's circulation has been at rest, the condition is especially distressing. In the evening, the pain becomes somewhat milder. In spite of the advanced aging process, it is often possible to attain relief, even freedom from pain, with therapeutic nourishment and with careful stimulation of the circulatory system by affusions over feet and arms and through mild massages. Gymnastic exercises with rapid head shifting and bends should be avoided by such patients. Good breathing and ample oxygen are important. Mental stimulation and enjoyment function as restorative aids. The *Bircher-Benner Salt-free Nutrition Plan,* Nash Publishing Co., Los Angeles, California, gives information on the particular food needs of aging people.

Heart Ailments

The headache of heart patients: The heart pumps blood unceasingly into all areas of the body. If it breaks down, certain areas are insufficiently supplied with oxygen and are burdened with metabolic waste. Inside the head, this creates the effect of a dull headache. With slowed beating of the heart, arterial blood mixes with venous blood. The patient's lips become blue and his face bluish. He cannot lie flat and, when he exerts himself, he complains of rapid heart beat, shortness of breath, a feeling of pressure on the heart and headache. The heart treatment, which includes a therapeutic diet as listed in *Handbook for Heart Patients* (to be published by Nash Publishing Co.), also cures the headache symptom.

Liver Disorders

Liver-function disorders after food poisoning, acute or chronic hepatitis, cirrhosis, or bile-duct infections also cause headaches through metabolic contamination. If the patient with a liver and gall bladder complaint enjoys a heavy, fatty meal, he is usually punished for it quickly, with headaches, a stuffed feeling, and nausea. Pain mounts, chiefly in the nape of the neck and the back of the head, spreading dully into the skull and the area of the crown. If the gall bladder were removed, the reserve bile would be lacking for larger amounts of food, and the so-called symptoms would then appear especially pronounced. After a heavy alcoholic drinking bout, a roaring head is a typical hangover symptom on waking up. This is a sign of the formation of waste in the liver that has hindered the work of detoxification and filtering as well as the manufacture of digestive juices. The treatment for the liver alone can cure headaches.*

Gastrointestinal Disorders

An organism which is metabolically overloaded for a long period of time very often suffers from chronic gastroenteritis. Although nutritionally deficient food may be consumed in large amounts, the body becomes deficient as a result of insufficient and defective assimilation. Subsequently, many side effects appear, that very often include headaches, neuralgic pains in different parts of the body, cramped capillary vessels and bad circulation, livid cheeks, red nose, and patchy reddening or pimples on the face. The head and its blood vessels are a delicate index to gastrointestinal overloading, inflammation, congestion, infection, decay, and fermentation. Obviously, these are significant warnings which indicate change and the need for therapeutic measures, so that the causes of the ailment can be removed.

---

*See *Nutrition Plan for Liver and Gall Bladder Patients* (soon to be published by Nash Publishing Corp.).

In order to cure the headache, the basic illness must be treated; excess acidity and overirritation of the stomach require a therapeutic diet. First in the cure, in any case, come rest and diet.

The slack, sluggish stomach, deficient in acid, is more difficult to put back in order, but here persistence will help attain this goal. A complete change in food intake, disciplined rebuilding exercise, walking, regulations of rest periods, and small amounts of food, well chewed, and particularly rich in fresh foods and enzymes, are necessary. Following this regimen will regulate the stomach and the headache will also disappear.

Any unusual conditions in the stomach area could cause headaches, as for example, diverticulum of the esophagus (an abnormal protruding pouch or sac), a hiatus hernia becoming chronically inflamed, a high-positioned cascade stomach, or postural changes through deformity. Such causes require special and also, if necessary, operative treatment, which then cures the headache at the same time.

Chronic and acute inflammation of the small intestine can also cause headaches. This is usually connected with liver, gall bladder, and pancreas disorders. An examination should also be made as to whether deformities, diverticulum, or displacement of neighboring organs might not be the underlying cause.

The colon is an old, well-known originator of headaches. Around the turn of the century, Arbuthnot Lane called it "the caldron of disease," and observed that the operative removal of the colon caused headaches, rheumatic illnesses, etc., to disappear. It subsequently became apparent, of course, that the same results can be attained better through food treatment, without removing the colon. Decay in the ascending colon, degeneration of the intestinal flora, and chronic constipation act as a focus of infection and a source of contamination to which the head reacts with a dull headache or even a migraine. The fact that a headache pill does not affect the basic cause is evident. Indeed, it only conceals the relationship, and leads to an impasse of chronic illness, as do most alleged shortcuts. The dietetic treatment of gastrointestinal diseases is thoroughly discussed in the *Bircher-Benner Nutrition Plan for Digestive Problems* (Nash Publishing Co.). The headache patient should familiarize himself with its contents.

Kidney Diseases

Chronic kidney diseases and nephrosclerosis, after nephritis and kidney poisoning from saturation with pain-killers, go along with headaches. Everyone today should know that pain-killers, stimulants, and sleeping pills taken regularly can cause severe kidney damage and prolonged headaches. In addicted persons, the discontinuance of pain-killers, as well as of alcohol, nicotine, etc., can also cause headaches, and many other symptoms. Only vigorous therapy and the strong will of the patient can prevent a recurrence of the illness if abstinence is attempted. Kidney failure (beginning uremia or eclampsia with pregnancy) exhibits a frontal headache as an outstanding symptom, swelling of the eyelids, numbness, and often nausea. This condition is dangerous. Every patient with kidney problems should see a physician. (*Handbook for Kidney and Bladder Patients,* soon to be published by Nash Publishing Co.).

Narrowing of Space in the Skull

Increased pressure in the skull cavity also causes headaches and is, in turn, caused by tumors, brain hemorrhages, brain concussions (swelling due to a blow on the skull which reaches the brain), and inflammations of the brain and its meninges (meningitis, encephalitis). This is so well known, that every sick person whose headache resists treatment for a day immediately thinks he has a brain tumor and asks his doctor for an explanation.

Meningitis and encephalitis are discussed on page 9. Tumor headaches have a special character and can probably be distinguished from other headaches by the doctor on the basis of special tests (eyeground examination, electroencephalogram, encephalograph, encephaloangiograph, and special blood tests). Should the findings be negative, the headache patient can stop worrying about a tumor.

Mental Illness

Mental illnesses can also occasionally begin with headaches that are easily diagnosed, since no anatomical cause can be found. Not until later, is it recognized that the patient's painful head sensations were advance sense disturbances and false physical sensations which later manifested themselves as mental illness. Today it is assumed that these symptoms arise, partially, from a disturbed metabolic equilibrium and, therefore, if recognized early enough can be effectively controlled. The deeper causes may be of an emotional or physiological origin, which a psychologist together with a physician can best explain.

Emotional Illness (See also p. 34.)

Emotional suffering, exhaustion, grief, overexertion, depression, and excessive mental work make the head act as a carrier of distressing memories, pains, pressure, numbness, and malaise—all transmitted into a headache. The depressed person often has a feeling of "leaden heaviness," "numbness of the head," or "dizziness." Only with difficulty does he overcome his feeling of aversion, forcing himself to do his daily work, while feeling overworked, and struggling steadfastly against his inner resistance and exhaustion. Very often, his head feels the pain and pressure, and his scalp is tight and sensitive to pressure. Since depression very often not only has emotional, but also physical causes and may stem from a disturbance of both physical and emotional equilibrium, this kind of headache must also be taken seriously. Disturbances of the liver, kidney, hormonal imbalance, anemia, acidemia, gout, etc., are physical reasons or tendencies which can lead to depression. They must be investigated and their physical background clarified.

A child who, because of his parents' ambition, attends a school which places too great a demand on his capabilities, can develop headaches in the conflict between "good intentions" and inner resistance. Loneliness, insurmountable obstacles, repressed hostility, and forced single-minded attempts to reach one's set goal ("butting one's head against a wall") can cause headaches. In this instance, the headache sufferer needs great understanding and patient, attentive talks. If the emotional relationships are understood, the cause of the headache is often removed and the headache as well.

Heat Stroke and Sunstroke

Overheating the body for long periods in hot rooms or in a hot climate can cause, in sensitive people, venous congestion in the head with debilitation of the blood vessels and impeded circulation. It can result in circulation breakdown and fainting spells with very severe headaches. However, with rest and cooling of the body, the disorders quickly fade away. Sunstroke results from excessive exposure to the sun, and the symptoms are the same as those of a brain concussion: local disturbance in the area of the head with swelling of the meninges, migraine headaches, nausea, and dizziness. Head pains are acute during sunning, fade very slowly, and can still leave behind a hypersensitivity to sunlight for weeks and months. It requires medical treatment and a rather long period of rest.

Frontal and Maxillary Sinuses

If strong frontal pressure unexpectedly occurs after a common head cold with discharge and neck pains, a frontal sinus inflammation (sinusitis) must be considered. These pains are concentrated in the region over the nasal bone and radiate slightly into the forehead and temporal region. They let up as soon as emptying of pus through the nose relieves the pressure. At the same time, the maxillary sinuses can become inflamed even without involving the frontal sinuses. The pain then becomes concentrated in the region on both sides of the nostrils and eyes and can also include the teeth. Nature offers us a large number of highly effective healing herbs of very varied uses, which, when combined with a therapeutic diet, rest, and treatment to bring down possible fever can lead to a cure, whereas antibiotics are used only in case of emergency since they breed resistant strains of bacteria and leave an exhausted patient to recover with difficulty. When a sinus inflammation (sinusitis) is suspected, a medical examination, including X-rays, is necessary and a number of possibilities should be considered. Often chronic tonsil inflammation (tonsilitis) or scattered infections in the teeth are the cause of pus formation in the sinuses and must first be cured, otherwise relapses and chronic headaches can be expected.

Infectious Diseases

Febrile diseases like pneumonia, viral diseases like measles, scarlet fever, mumps, and infantile paralysis, usually begin with headaches and often lead to toxic meningitis (meningism). If an infectious disease also causes striking, unbearable headaches, genuine meningitis must be considered and immediate medical help obtained. Cool neck compresses should be applied until the doctor comes. The room should be darkened and absolute quiet provided. With the rise in temperature from fever, an increased flow of blood penetrates into the blood vessels and meninges. This causes pressure and pain. It happens that a headache is the only symptom of pneumonia or other febrile disease in the beginning. This is a warning signal that enables an early diagnosis.

Tuberculosis

It is well known that lung and abdominal tuberculosis patients suffer from headaches due to the effect of bacterial toxins. Less known, perhaps, is the fact that "cured" persons who have returned from a fattening tuberculosis diet and have reacted to the fattening diet with liver and intestinal damage, retain their headaches even after their return. Patients treated with high doses of antibiotics during infectious diseases subsequently suffer from a disturbed intestinal flora with dyspepsia, enteritis, and headaches. After heavy meals, sharp spices, and sweets, they react very quickly with a headache.

Accidents

Patients in accidents involving brain concussion or skull injury can be left with headaches for years, in case of insufficient healing. For this reason, the doctor prescribes a long period of bedrest after a brain concussion, often for several weeks, and complete care of the head. What appears to be a slight accident can also cause dizziness, headaches, amnesia, or short fainting spells, nausea, or vomiting. These are symptoms which fade away with complete rest.

Eyes

Constant straining of the eyes, continuous night work, and working in glaring, harsh, or insufficient light, from a poor source and in narrow spaces, place too great a burden on the capacity of the eye muscles to adjust and cause irritation of the blood vessels of the eye. Looking through a microscope for a long period or reading small print for a long time can result in not only painful, itching, and swollen eyes, but can also cause frontal and temporal headaches. After any activity that strains the eyes, it helps to relax them by rubbing them gently with the hands and fully loosening the eye muscles, then looking at something far away, preferably something green. In the case of unidentified aching of the eye that comes on as attacks, one should seriously consider the possibility of increased pressure on the eyeball (glaucoma), and an ophthalmologist should be consulted early. Vitamin A is important during growth for the healthy development and continuing health of the eyes.

Neck and Cervical Vertebrae

A neck pain (cervical syndrome) is another form of headache. It begins as a gentle drawing pain at the nape of the neck and can cause a feeling as of tightly stretched wires on one or both sides of the neck. It moves from the neck into the skull and on its way can cause "crushing" pains in the shoulder region and neck and even in the forehead.

These headaches are above all, of a rheumatic nature, and are caused by deposits in muscles, tendons, and fatty tissue, which exert pressure on the blood vessels and nerves. They cause muscular constriction that makes the patient feel as if a heavy load were lying on his neck. The person who sits stooped over at work or whose head position is bent over in relation to the spine because of poor posture ever since he went to school, in later years often suffers from such rheumatic changes also affecting the vertebrae of the neck and causing the small joints between the cervical vertebrae to swell up and become deformed. A child carries his spine (cervical vertebrae) proud and straight over his hips. But on learning to write and carry a schoolbag, or, standing afraid in front of strict parents and teachers, his posture too often becomes stooped, laterally and lopsidedly, so that cervical vertebrae are deformed. In addition, calcium and vitamin deficiencies appear (from lack of sun), so that the vertebrae are also weakened by changes caused by these deficiencies. Later in life, this also causes cervical arthrosis which can hamper the development of individual nerve centers resulting in severe neuralgia. Many pains in the neck, skull, and arms are caused by rheumatically altered cervical vertebrae and can be cured only if they receive special care. In addition to the general treatment of basic rheumatic illness through a regulated therapy (*Bircher-Benner Nutrition Plan for Rheumatism and Arthritis,* Nash Publishing Co.), connective tissue massages, affusions promoting circulation, and compresses, stretching, often shortwave treatments, and also chiropractic treatment can help provided the condition is not too far advanced. Heat has also proven to be helpful. With all treatments, subsequent correct posture and movement is of the utmost importance (see neck exercises, p. 153).

Neuralgia

The neuralgic headache is a sharp piercing, nerve-headache (neuralgia). It appears suddenly with a change in weather and during certain seasons, as pain behind the ear that spreads over the jaw, forehead, and eyes, usually on one side. It seems to disappear while resting, only to flare up again even more suddenly. This neuralgic headache is an extremely annoying but, fortunately, rare illness. It can affect different nerve branches. Best known is trigeminus neuralgia, which branches out below the ear to the temples, eyes, and cheeks. The occipital nerve in the back of the head and the nerve centers above and below the orbital cavities can also cause neuralgic pains of the first order. At times, these attacks occur repeatedly for days or weeks, similar to the well-known neuritis of the upper arm (brachial neuritis) or of the sciatic nerve.

The cause can lie in viral illnesses, a center of infection in the teeth, tonsils, intestine, gall bladder, frontal and maxillary sinuses, etc., or in damage by metabolic poisons. The nerve can be damaged as a result of the effect of a chill (cold) or by pressure of a tumor within the head. The cause of head neuralgia is often physical or mental exhaustion, which follows upon using up one's reserves and a resultant deficiency in the Vitamin B complex.

Shingles (Herpes Zoster)

If nerve branches in the neck and head region are attacked, shingles also begins with neuralgic headaches. We are now dealing with a particular viral infection of the nerve center, which needs intensive treatment. Other virus groups, influenza, and festerings can cause head neuralgia, and, in addition, also alcohol, certain drugs, and diabetes.

Because of this variety of possible causes, quick medical diagnosis is desirable and, if necessary, special medical care. Large injections of Vitamin B, shortwave treatments, hot baths, raw-diet periods, and elimination of the center of infection are decisively important for facilitating a cure. A light diet is important that is easy on the liver and rich in raw food, and that bypasses heated fats, snacks of sweets, excess protein, alcohol, and other irritants, for the liver plays a central role as an organ of detoxification in all toxic-inflammatory diseases.

Allergies

Allergenic headaches: allergic reactions indicate a diseased, overtaxed organism. It accompanies a long prehistory, often including an inherited damaged constitution. Forms of allergic illnesses are: asthma, hay fever, edema, eczema, hives (urticaria), allergic diarrhea, and dyspepsia after consuming indigestible food. There are also emotional allergies. Common to all allergies is an excessive reaction to an insignificant stimulant. Most allergic reactions involve headaches, usually of the character of a migraine (see page 28). Almost all people who are allergic have a markedly deficient diet, with an excess of fat and animal protein, too much salt, many irritants, too much sugar, too many roasts and cooked products, and too much alcohol. They also have a disturbed acid-alkali equilibrium in their blood and body tissue.

An allergic thrust, expressed in a variety of symptoms—which also includes migraines—means a constriction of capillaries, water flow into the tissue, and swelling of the mucous membrane or skin in different places on the body (nose, bronchia, crotch and armpits, eyes, skin). Centers of infection can function as a constant irritant, as do excitement, anger, and haste. Headaches are almost always part of the syndrome of allergic patients. Upon overcoming the allergy, the headache that almost always accompanies it disappears. Asthma, hay fever, and migraines often alternate in the same person. Cortisone is often given today, with sudden success in the remission of symptoms, but without healing. Healing requires a change in the condition of the tissue, detoxification, discharge, and lasting freedom from the tendency to exaggerated response. Success must come from the inside, out. It is not dramatically attained all at once, but it will bring lasting freedom (see chapter on diets for allergic patients in the Bircher-Benner cookbook *Eating Your Way to Health* published by Penguin Books, Inc.

Two Headache Patients

1. A seventeen-year-old girl suffered from daily headaches, fatigue, aversion to work, and depression. This condition had been worsening for two years, and became so advanced that, in spite of her youth, she had to take headache tablets several times a week. One morning she could not go to school because she had a fainting spell followed by dizziness. Her mother sent her to the doctor.

The girl was pale, had swollen features, and a bad complexion. As a high school student, she had an overcrowded schedule, from 7 A.M. to 6 P.M., including private lessons and homework, and did not go to bed until 10 P.M., rising in the morning with quite an effort, gulping down her breakfast, and flying to school. Industrious and conscientious as she was, she hardly came in contact with the fresh air. Her mother provided her with "strengthening" food: meat, eggs, soup, milk, white bread, and pudding—almost no fresh fruit or salad. The result: chronic constipation, aggravated by "simply-not-having-the-time" during the morning rush. This behavior causes countless young people to suffer from enteroplegia. Headaches always show up as a result. They begin in the morning and complicate work during the day. What to do? Exams were approaching and under no circumstances could she fail. Night work and fatigue increased, and her intestine no longer worked at all. She therefore took headache tablets and laxatives more and more frequently. They produced a peculiar, dizzying, floating alertness in which unsteadiness and a feeling of unreality were alternately mingled. She also began to smoke a few cigarettes in the morning. This calmed her down and allowed her intestine to work. Then, finally, fainting spells occurred, which brought her to the doctor. Findings: anemia, vertigo, and fainting spells are the typical expression of drug and nicotine poisoning. Chronic constipation, poor circulation, and a bad complexion are typical signs of vitamin and mineral deficiency, which especially begins to show its effects in puberty. The results: headaches. What can be done?

The way was clear: she immediately switched over to fresh food, three times daily and before every meal, followed by whole-wheat bread, ground-wheat mash, and green leafy salad. The intestinal activity which improved through this quickly relieved the headaches. A scheduling of the day was devised whereby regular amounts of sunlight and exercise in fresh air was made possible; in addition, dry brushing, affusions, and skin care. During holidays, she was able to sunbath and perspire. In due course, skin and head were completely restored to health. The most difficult part of the job was of freeing the young organism from its dependency on nicotine and pills, to which it had become addicted. Dizziness and depression still persisted for a rather long time and complicated the task. The patient had to be encouraged, advised, and guided in maintaining her willpower. Success gave her new vitality and successful self-control gave her new self-confidence. She was successful in breaking her bad habits because she was still young, intelligent, and sensible. She truly wanted to be cured and free from illness with all her might.

The way looks simple, but it is not easy to travel. The struggle for recovery, especially in the beginning, requires inner strength on the part of the patient and understanding on the part of his companions. Such a victory, however, makes for joy and satisfaction and develops a mature personality. The experience of transforming one's own life through one's own power without the help of drugs, and of being healed in this way, is unforgettable.

2. A pale, slender, tired-looking woman in her early 40s was undergoing clinical treatment for chronic headaches which had not responded to treatment. As the wife of a businessman, she had social obligations in addition to running her household and took frequent trips, during which she ate in hotels. As a well-groomed and ready spouse, she has to endure such occasions without showing fatigue. She is enchanting and fulfills her task with unfailing conscientiousness and self-discipline. She expects the same from her children and friends.

This patient was also a fragile woman. She was frequently ill as a child. She had to fight against increasing exhaustion and make more and more of an effort to save face. As a young girl, she suffered a pulmonary glandular tuberculosis and eclampsia (convulsions) and kidney failure with high blood pressure during the birth of her third child. She has been suffering from anemia for years.

She has childhood memories of her mother, who died early. She was very fragile, suffered incessantly from headaches, and took pills at every meal (the children had to bring them home from the drugstore). It is no wonder that pill-gulping also became an obvious recourse for the daughter when headaches began to torture her more and more frequently. These headaches began soon after she had undergone treatment for tuberculosis, which entailed a fattening diet and rest. They began to attack her in the morning on waking up, especially after upsetting days or after festive occasions, at rather large intervals at first, then more and more frequently. Finally, a heavy-feeling forehead, drawing pains in her neck, and maddening head pains were her daily morning greeting. Nevertheless, she had to get through the day and do her duty, which she did well, yes, even brilliantly. No one had to know that it was done with more and more pills.

Six to ten pills a day! When Mrs. N. came to the clinic, she was so far-gone that even that many pills no longer helped. In addition, constipation persisted and menstruation was irregular, painful, and linked with increasing headaches. Investigation showed advanced, threatening kidney inflammation and anemia—classic signs of painkiller poisoning. Depression also appeared and constant loss of weight and high blood pressure. The headaches were rooted in her genetic make-up reinforced by her mother's example as well as in the forced metabolic overloading caused by the fattening diet and rest in the tuberculosis sanitorium, in chronic constipation, and dependence on painkillers which had led to kidney damage and anemia.

The treatment, in this case also, was a painful road for the patient to travel, but she traveled it bravely, conscious of the danger which threatened her life through kidney failure (uremia) and of responsibility to her family. Juice fast days, raw food periods several times a week, daily bed rest with mild, warm baths and compresses, brief massages in the kidney region, massage of connective tissue in the zones of the intestine and kidney, showering at various temperatures, dry brushing of the badly perfused skin to stimulate circulation and autogenous training for complete relaxation were subsequently carried out. Instead of the headache pill for pain, she used hot neck and back compresses. She had regular conversations with her doctor for explaining cause, effect, and remedy.

Success came slowly. Blood quality improved, as did the functioning of kidneys and intestine. Weight gradually increased, in spite of a small amount of food. During the three weeks of treatment in the clinic, progress was not so difficult. It was different at home, where she found herself faced with her old household habits. Bed rest and a raw diet alleviated the headaches that broke out again with exertion as much as possible. Meat, fish, coffee, tea, and salt caused prompt relapses and were therefore strictly avoided.

In the time that followed, the patient's condition was checked at quarterly intervals by her doctor. If she took drugs, high blood pressure, kidney breakdown, and increased anemia immediately appeared. After one year, her condition was largely standardized for the first time. Mrs. N. has put on weight. She appears to be doing very well and is again in high spirits.

The children, who because of their sick mother were becoming sickly, are also doing very well. One of them was already inclined to have chronic headaches, and had attracted attention in school by being too conscientious. He is now visibly recuperating.

Summary

There are very different kinds of headaches and very different causes, the commonest being the poisoning of the organism, diminishing health through alienation of the natural order of physical and mental life. The first step on a headache patient's way to recovery is: return to a healthy life-style with high quality but small quantities of nourishment, daily physical exercise, correct posture, resolution of conflicts, tension, and despondency. It is important to study the life of a person afflicted with headaches and to find out the conditions under which the headache began. Has it existed since childhood? Did the mother or father suffer from it? Is an infectious disease the cause? A liver, stomach, or intestinal disorder? Did it begin on the occasion of a large formal banquet or after a period of physical or nervous stress? Did it appear in connection with a severe head cold?

Mental illness is often the main cause of headaches. As a carrier of thoughts and a mediator of mental power, the head must be kept clean and clear. A dusty electric bulb cannot shine clearly. The head is a very sensitive index instrument of all disorderly processes in the organism. For this reason, research and treatment of headaches are very important.

II. Migraines

Causes and Meaning of Migraines

A migraine is also a headache, but with very peculiar symptoms. It must be discussed here thoroughly, because it is one of the severest forms of all headaches and is considered more and more threatening today. It is different from a simple headache in intensity, in its sudden occurrence in usually ordinary circumstances, in the fact that the pain alternately attacks on only one side of the head (hemicrania), and that it is frequently accompanied by nausea and vomiting. It is a convulsive illness of an allergic character and usually begins in youth, frequently fading away in old age.

A migraine is a disease which attacks countless people suddenly, often as an awful scourge, and in a wide range, from a slight morning headache to deep depression lasting for several days. It keeps them from functioning in more or less ordinary circumstances.

The week-end migraine is notorious. It occurs almost exactly at the moment when the patient changes over from the nervous tension of his weekly work to the week-end or to vacation time. Just when he is letting go, when he sleeps longer in the morning, and changes the rhythm of day and night, a conversion of the vegetative (nutritional and growth functions) nervous system begins; then the organism catches up with what is lacking and begins a "cleaning" process with more or less dramatic effort. This cleaning process can be experienced in very different ways: simple exhaustion, pains in the limbs, distending infections, lumbago, and depression previously suppressed by activity in work and by drugs, can simultaneously break out all over. In the course of this, the body tries, in fits and starts, to get rid of all collected poisons, deposits, and residue. The most emphatic drama of purification is a migraine.

People respond, in very different ways, to their body and its language. One kind of person grieves about his "unmerciful destiny" and fights the constant misfortune of ruined leisure time, another person looks for and finds the cause and effect, goes "to the heart of the matter," learns and understands. He recovers by acting out of knowledge, and matures from the experience gained from healthy "fault and atonement." Overcoming a migraine puts one through the school of suffering and self-knowledge and thereby brings great human gain.

A migraine is almost always curable on condition that causative therapy is consistently followed.

What is meant by a migraine? An intensive headache that occurs on one side of the head, frequently changing sides, usually at regular intervals. It often begins in the early morning hours, between 1 and 5 A.M., especially after days of intensive mental or physical strain, but often even without any apparent cause. In women, a migraine often seems to occur in relation to menstruation, usually occurring immediately before or after the onset of the menstrual cycle. In patients who are sensitive to weather, it occurs with almost mathematical certainty at the first sign of an atmospheric front bringing a strong sudden change, as in the case of a spring storm, cold winds, chill, or snow. It then occurs usually 1 to 2 days before the change in weather, just as if it had a presentiment of their arrival. In the case of migraines determined on the basis of weather conditions, it is assumed that a change in the electric tension of the atmosphere is the cause. In a number of investigations, it was found that an atmospheric charge of negative ions works against migraines, whereas one with a positive charge promotes migraines (bio-climatic).

Various methods of astute observation of migraines contribute to our understanding them: First, 1 to 2 days of striking good health, energy, good and abundant appetite and bowel movements, clear and copious urine. Immediately before the migraine: Nervousness, disturbed sleep, overstimulated appetite, desire for sharp spices, constipation, reduction in the amount of urine, rise in blood pressure. At the moment the migraine occurs, a shift takes place to the other extreme: Great need for rest, drop in blood pressure, desire to avoid noise and light, headache, incapacity to think and eat, nausea, stomach cramps. The first prior signs of a migraine are characterized by a kind of warning known as an "aura": Twitching of the eye, buzzing in the ears, sensitivity to heat and cold, dizziness, occasionally impediments in speech and hearing with an effort to concentrate and an inability to find words, extreme itchiness with feelings similar to slight paralysis. These symptoms all correspond to constrictions in blood vessels and are related to symptoms usually preceding an epileptic fit.

In the migraine attack itself, along with the piercing pain over the orbital cavities, the forehead, and one side of the skull and into the neck, there is sensitivity to light and noise, and especially nausea, often with serious vomiting of bile and clogging of the esophagus, combined with thirst. First dark, concentrated urine, then large amounts of clear urine. Many patients turn pale grey or yellow. Nausea and bilious vomiting, feelings of despair and despondency, freezing, fear, dizziness, and occasionally fainting spells alternate with each other. The attack usually lasts 12 to 24 hours and sometimes longer.

This condition can bring anybody to despair, and the fearful patient seeks to prevent it with all possible means and reaches for strong drugs at the slightest warning sign or before the beginning of the actual crisis. As the migraine attack fades, urine and stool again return to normal. In addition, there is a desire for care, purification, avoiding exertion and stress. Stage before the migraine: Sympatheticotonia (overactivity of the central nervous system). Stage during the migraine: Vagotonia (exaggerated stimulation of the vagus nerve). Purpose of cure: Equalizing the extremes, resulting in general relief. Today, migraines are no longer thought of as a disease, but a search is being made for a way to free the body of the necessity of using a migraine as a "catastrophic remedy." The cause will be found and there will no longer be any need to drug it.

Migraines can be suppressed by many kinds of tricks, as with coffee or tea in light cases, or by filling the stomach, or by taking pills. However, these maneuvers can never prevent the attack from recurring after the so-called "respite" has ended. It may then perhaps be delayed artifically one or more times, but when these remedies no longer work, the pain breaks out even more violently. Since every symptom is significant only in the context of the whole person it is also necessary here to investigate the meaning of entire attack, for only the knowledge of cause and meaning can open the way to recovery.

In the first phase, a migraine consists of constriction of blood vessels in certain zones of the head. In this way, the circulation of blood in the fine capillaries within the scalp, meninges, and cortex is retarded. This is the warning phase. The migraine patient turns pale, tense, and has the warning symptoms described on page 21 ("cold migraine"). The second phase or actual migraine then develops into blood-vessel dilation, especially of the capillaries, and this congestion causes the characteristic tense pain which goes along with reddening and a feeling of warmth in the head ("hot migraine"). The pain as well as the subsequent dilation are hypersensitive reactions (allergies) to fluctuations in the metabolism. The change from pale grey in the prestage to congestive reddening during the attack is typical of migraines; chill in the beginning and heatwaves during the attack.

Metabolism and the Vegetative System

An organism which has to struggle against the results of decades of incorrect nutrition and is overloaded with metabolic wastes, insidious infections, and poisons is in an overstimulated condition that makes it react abnormally to variations in its internal operation and to changes in the environment. If the metabolic error becomes advanced, then a warning device goes into operation for relieving tension, and commencing a detoxification and healing process. The vegetative nervous system, our powerful regulatory nervous system with its paired design of sympathetic and vagus nerves, goes into action. At the beginning of our century, in 1904, the English physician, Alexander Haig, had already observed that he could reduce severe migraines with a diet that was low in meat and salt, and fully overcome them with a strictly vegetable diet that was rich in fresh food. He was the first doctor to recognize metabolic disturbance and hyperacidity of the blood from purine as the basis of convulsive illnesses and particularly of migraines, and, consequently, he was able to overcome it with diet. The accuracy of his observations and results has again been fully brought to light in the course of modern research (see pp. 41-46).

But let us return to the vegetative system and its regulatory function: If the sympathetic nervous system predominates, the body is in a suitable condition to perform work and to enter into contact and conflict with the outside world, expend energy, and build up reserves. The metabolism is in a state of hyperacidity and not in a position to carry out its functions of detoxification. Such a condition is normal during the day, if it is limited to a few hours at a time. If, however, it is unduly expanded, especially into the night, then the alleviating and detoxifying adjustment from the effect of the vagus for relaxation, sleep, and rest is lacking. Such a lag in adjustment arises with professional and social stress and with stress from overindulgence and stimulants, if they are prolonged. If suitable rest periods are lacking, although they should occur at intervals during the course of a regulated day, if the naturally needed period of night sleep is lacking or is long delayed by staying awake at night and sleeping during the day, there will be damage to organs, insidious bacterial poisoning (in liver, bladder, tonsils, renal pelvis, gastrointestinal system, teeth and gums, abdominal organs, etc.), and the equilibrium in the vegetative nervous system will thus be more and more disturbed. The time for conserving and increasing energy, drainage, detoxification, restoration of hyperalkalinity, and rest is taken away from the organism and with it, the possibility of going to work purified, strengthened, and freshly charged after a night of thorough rest. In emergencies, a body produces unsuspected energy for a short period, but it will break down over a long period. An environment filled with tension, frequently changing weather, intoxication from nicotine, alcohol, metabolic poisons, and drugs which invade the vegetative system (appetite depressants, sedatives, tranquilizers, stimulants, laxatives, etc.), often decisively promote disturbance in the vegetative equilibrium.

The inclination to restrain stress and overstimulation leaves a person too little room and time for relaxation, purification, and accumulation—if he unconsciously resists—and prevents the restoration of equilibrium between the expenditure and the new load of energy. The body remains too long and too much in sympatheticotonia and does not give vagotonia enough time to fully do its work. Thus, dangerous residue collects in body and mind and there are only two ways out of this: either the way into sickness or a return to an orderly life-style. If the suffering is strong, so is the will to recover from it.

Considered in this light, a migraine is none other than the organism's attempt to force necessary relief and equilibrium on the way to vagotonia in the form of an overwhelming catastrophe. A migraine is not an illness in itself, as we now understand the word, but the spur to a spontaneous maneuver for recovery and, therefore, requires attention, observation, and very precise examination of the total condition preceding it. On the other hand, if migraines are combated as a disease, and suppressed with painkillers, the result cannot be considered a cure, but a strengthening and rigidification of the disorder, that dangerous condition which Dr. Bircher-Benner called "incipient disease." The result will be that new migraine attacks will occur more and more frequently.

It is necessary to draw a picture of a migraine patient's metabolic condition. In a blood-serum analysis for the period when no headaches exist, migraine patients often show high uric-acid values (acidosis), which decline in the premigraine phase with increasing backflow into the tissue. In the process, alkali reserves decline. Immediately after the attack, there is a rapid increase of uric acid in the blood serum. The uric acid has flowed back out of the tissue into the blood stream, increasing to astonishingly high density, which may last for a few hours. Urea, creatinine, salt, and other metabolic products react similarly to uric acid. Capillaries show constriction before a migraine, dilation with backflow during a migraine, and normalization and equal flow of blood after a migraine.

In 1927, Dr. Gaensslen substantiated that capillary constriction took place when hyperacidity of the blood lasted several days, as in the case of excessive consumption of meat by the test subjects (students), and a recovery of the capillaries occurred after converting to a predominantly fresh food diet. In the acidosis phase, these test subjects very often reacted with migrainelike pains. Those metabolic products, which had to flow from spaces between cells and cell tissue and from the lymph stream through the blood and kidneys, for excretion, become congested until the tolerable limit of stress is exceeded, then forcing a convulsive relief. This corresponds to the picture of a migraine and can be observed as a classic curve, as described above. Our clinical observations and modern medical research confirm this.

The Migraine Person

A migraine usually occurs for the first time between the ages of 15 and 35. Women suffer from it more often than men. As one would suppose, hormonal variations and the correspondingly sensitive condition of equilibrium of their vegetative nervous system is involved. Very few women, many fewer than men, have the opportunity to relax after professional or household work, or both, if they are to provide a good atmosphere for their family and always stand "at the ready." Women tend not to relax, because of an overriding sense of responsibility and need for perfection, and are thus more inclined to suppress their migraines with drugs at their first appearance. As a result, dependency on painkillers is very often observed in women. This, in turn, causes headaches and migraines, like intoxication itself.

Migraine people are usually delicately built, graceful, slim, and active people, with resolute and nervous personalities. Their faces bear an expression of full concentration and strong self-discipline. Their skin is usually pale, often visibily tender. Their thoughts are sharply outlined, with a basic intellectual attitude and inclination to come to logical conclusions. They do not allow themselves to be overcome by emotion, and easily and spontaneously suppress emotional excitement with an iron will. Behind this there is usually sensitivity, vulnerability, insecurity, and often carefully hidden depression. Their peripheral circulation is not good, their capillaries tend to constrict and are seen as a corkscrew shape under a microscope, their blood circulates slowly, hands and feet are pale bluish and cold, in winter they frequently have white fingers or chilblain. In order to counteract this chill, they tend instinctively to hyperkinesia and are constantly active; this leads to an exaggerated performance drive accompanied by nervousness and agression. Like their circulation, their digestion first tends toward constriction, their intestine to spastic constipation followed by dilation and diarrhetic counterreactions.

Convulsive Diseases Equivalent to Migraines

There are a number of related convulsive diseases based on the same basic metabolic condition and displaying the same typical variations in blood and urine. Thus, for example, regular onsets of speech impediments, stomach, intestinal, and gall bladder colic ("abdominal migraine"), coronary constrictions (angina pectoris), and other bronchial cramps with asthma or even epilepticlike fits and absentias. Attacks of rheumatism, lumbago, and stiff necks also go along with variations in metabolism. These crisislike convulsive illnesses give the impression of being threatening conditions, but they are, at first, purely functional, which means that they are subdued after the attack fades away. They recur frequently, however, over the years and thus gradually do damage and pave the way for later severe organic diseases in old age. Frequent seizures of stomach, intestinal, and gall bladder colic, leave behind a tendency to ulcers, swellings, formation of stones and inflammation; to diverticulum in the intestine, to thrombosis and infarct in the coronary blood vessels; and, frequently, constriction of the blood vessels of the brain making its appearance later in sudden attacks, etc. The form this disturbance of the bodies' metabolic stability will take to make one sick, depends on hereditary predisposition, on diet and environmental damage, on the condition of the body, and one's sex. In this connection, the endocrine glands also play an important role: the pituitary gland (hypophysis cerebri), thyroid gland, adrenal glands, and the gonads are involved with each other in constant interaction in regulating the metabolism. Emotional behavior—relations with parents at home, emotional upsets, arguments with friends, loss of self-confidence, unfulfilled wishes for power and possessions, and many others—can prepare the ground for a migraine.

The Case History of Migraine Patients

If a case history of a migraine patient were thoroughly researched before his illness, approximately the following chain of events would be apparent from youth on: A difficult pregnancy of the mother with strong nausea and an incorrect diet; possibly experiences of shock, depression, insecurity and discord at home; an unhealthy life-style for a long period, even before puberty; the habit of eating sweets, a fattening diet, a tendency to gastroenteritis; various allergic reactions in later life: an extremely unhealthy diet with increasing use of irritants (caffeine, alcohol, nicotine, salt, chocolate), white flour, sweets, and other processed foods, lack of fresh food, nervous overstimulation, psychic stress from tense professional, social, and family conditions, overexertion.

The overemphasis on intellectual development in schools, today, and a lack of exercise and sleep, coupled with prolonged fears about grades and examinations are dangerous for the autonomic system, (especially for those with a tendency to have convulsive diseases). The detoxifying function of the liver and the function of the endocrine glands, and especially the gonads, are interrelated. They strongly influence the autonomic (respiration, circulation, digestion, etc.) system. Both can break down and mutually weaken each other if the metabolism is overloaded and if there is a deficiency of minerals, vitamins, enzymes, and other vital nutritional materials. If the foundation is damaged in a young person merely an acute illness or an emotional disturbance, to which he has already been exposed in puberty, is needed to cause the first attack of migraine. It is tragic for such a patient to be labeled with the embarrassing diagnosis, "psychosomatic migraine," and the problem is consequently shelved. Psychic causes must also be taken seriously as the cause of physical illness. The remedy is clearly indicated. In a young person, the prospects for healing are good if living habits are reordered on an emotional as well as a physical basis, and if the new resolutions are decisively and persistently put into effect.

In female migraine patients, as stated previously, an attack is frequently linked to menstruation, as the menses favor the elimination of metabolic residue and liquid in the tissues. If the attacks are later suppressed with headache remedies, vagus nerve depressants, and stimulants, they increase in strength and frequency and also occur between menstrual periods. Before menstruation, women are tense, overexcited, and their bodies swell and retain water. They sleep late and restlessly and are constipated. With the recurrence of menstruation, a migraine breaks out with a large flow of urine, partially with profuse bleeding. During menopause, the tendency to migraines slowly fades away.

Early and Late Migraine

Early cases of migraines can almost always be cured. If the illness is very far advanced, however, a cure is not always possible, but improvement probably is, as long as liver, blood vessels, and other organs have not suffered massive, irreparable damage. This ever-recurring constriction is often the cause of high blood pressure in later life. Accompanying inflammations of liver tissue and bile duct often need thorough care. Very often the stomach is inflamed, the mucous membrane is irritated, stomach-acid secretion is reduced or is completely absent, so that the food remains too long in the stomach, decomposes, and poisons the blood. A migraine patient, however, who has already suffered for years and has many despondent hours behind him, will assist in the cure with great energy and patience and as soon as possible, for he knows what is necessary to be free of this evil. A "beginner" often does not realize the significance of causative treatment and later reaches for the tricks and ways mentioned above, which delay the attacks somewhat, and complicate the problem.

Focal Infection and Allergy (see also p. 13)

A serious problem is formation of *focal bacterial infection* and the allergic reaction which easily develops on top of it. This infection is given a strong assist by the body's weakening resistance that results from an unhealthy life-style.

Tooth decay because of insufficient care makes possible infections in the gums and the roots of the teeth. Additional bacterial centers of infection might be formed in the tonsils, sinuses, bronchia, chronically inflamed, with bronchiectasis (enlargement of the bronchia), abdominal organs (in men, prostatitis, in women, adnexitis, cervixitis). In the case of chronic constipation or inflammation, the intestine and its appended organs—liver, gall bladder, and pancreas—become particular centers of poisoning through the insidious flow of bacteria or their toxins. The organism is placed in a state of continual fighting and irritation by a focal infection, and hypersensitivity (allergy) can finally develop from this condition. A migraine allergy can also be the result of a focal infection, and a slight stimulant, a head cold, overexertion, insignificant excitement, a rich meal, a bite of lobster, a spoonful of mayonnaise, or a sip of alcohol can then, apparently, be enough to cause an attack in which the delicate network of nerves surrounding the capillaries are displaced in allergic irritation and constriction. Once it has become allergic, the organism reacts more and more frequently in the form of other allergies, so that, in the end, fears of the forbidden meal's triggering mechanisms "shoot up like toadstools."

Testing the body for allergies, that is, for substances that cause allergic reactions like rashes, asthma, hay fever, migraines, abdominal cramps, and diarrhea, can furnish valuable information and be useful in starting treatment. The value of these tests must not be overestimated, however. Treatment must transform the organism to such an extent that it shows no allergic reactions at all. This state is reached only when the causes responsible for the allergy are uprooted. A therapeutic diet and a healthy way of life are the means by which the diseased body can be brought back into equilibrium. In addition, focuses of infection must be eliminated and the body's resistance increased. The patient must be informed of these relationships in detail.

The Intestinal Source

In the case of migraines, an intestinal infection most often plays the role of the focal point. There is hardly a migraine patient who does not complain of chronic constipation with malaise, a sated feeling, cramps, gas, and belching. There is hardly a migraine patient who does not complain of the indigestibility of various foods. The ascending colon becomes flaccid and loose from constipation, and many blood vessels lead from it to the liver. In the appendix, that partial blind alley, cellulose digestion and the activity of the normal intestinal bacterial flora should again go into operation. The result is the stimulation of colonic peristalsis. If a fresh diet, rich in vital materials, with its abundance of enzymes and cellulose and their ability to regenerate the intestinal environment again and again, has been missing from the diet for years, the intestine becomes exhausted and flaccid and forms an environment of decay and fermentation. This degenerated environment works like a focus of infection and poisons the whole organism with toxins that penetrate through the intestinal wall into the blood. If the bacterial flora in the intestine degenerate, the intestinal mucosa become inflamed and permeable to toxins and bacteria. Bacterial colitis, for example, is caused in this way; it is a flooding of the body with degenerate strains of intestinal bacteria that damage liver and bile ducts, kidneys, and the circulatory and nervous systems. These bacteria can also lead to abnormal resistance reactions, including migraines. From the colon, the infection rises into the small intestine, and from there into liver ducts and gall bladder, and also, frequently, into the pancreas. The liver weakens in its detoxification capacity and bile production, and in turn, constipation and metabolic stress increase.

The patient must understand clearly, that at that time a radical interference with his living habits has become absolutely unavoidable—perhaps for the rest of his life. They must be totally revised. Unless will and ability are strong enough, it is better that the patient should not start this treatment. Lasting recovery cannot be achieved half-heartedly.

Prevention and Treatment of Migraines

Diet

Effective migraine treatment begins with a knowledge of nutrition as the basis for all further measures. A high-quality diet, as is well known, is effective against inflammation, detoxifies, relieves, dehydrates, increases resistance, and regenerates. It stabilizes the autonomic system, which reacts very sensitively to disturbances in the acid-alkali equilibrium and is the first to suffer from the effects of a focus of infection, intoxication, or exhaustion. A high-quality, well-balanced diet, its natural consistency untouched, relieves the liver, stimulates the flow of bile and digestive secretion, works against decay and fermentation in the intestine in general, and assures the necessary, oxygen-free environment needed in the intestine for normal digestion. The fact that this cannot be achieved by headache pill or the popular spasmolytic-ergot remedy, or through antiallergenic drugs needs no further explanation.

Just as in other matters, genuine strength and value lie in simplicity. Thus, something so simple as plain fresh raw food takes a key position. It has the ability to regenerate the intestinal and liver functions. During an attack, the migraine patient will instinctively reach for fresh vegetables and fruit juices, fresh natural vegetable broth and herb tea, mineral water—mild, simple tastes—and will decline anything processed, concentrated, and hard to digest as well as stimulants, fats, and strong spices. He reduces his amount of food to a minimum, while liver, bile, blood, and tissue recuperate. Only one desire prevails: rest during the internal struggle; no harsh light, no conversation, no loud noise, no absorption of food.

The wonderful gift of instinct, which expresses itself in such a way, unfortunately again abandons the body after the attack is over, just as it has generally been lost in the course of the progress of civilization. If a migraine attack is suppressed (with drugs) before its outbreak, this instinct-regulated short recovery also does not take place.

In addition to adopting a new diet, clinical care and supervision are often necessary in the beginning for accelerating detoxification and protecting the liver: Liver drainage with a duodenal probe, possibly herb enemas, and doses of vitamins and minerals, temporarily, are all things that support the course of deep-rooted therapeutic treatment. If tests show that bacterial infectious causes are foremost, immunization treatment can also be of help after removal of the focus of infection. A typical example is the patient who has had tuberculosis, scrophula, jaundice, or gall bladder disease and becomes ill with a migraine (allergic) after a fattening diet.

Vacation or more relaxed working hours are needed during the first stage of changing eating and living habits. This is a possible way to begin: once or twice, a one quart camomile enema. Seven to 14 days of strict raw diet, accompanied also by fresh-juice fasts, provided a doctor controls the diet. (People who have had experience with diets can carry them out alone.) Then, a raw diet with small supplements of cooked food consisting of whole-wheat bread and potatoes cooked in their jackets, but the diet must still consist of 80% to 90% fresh food. After this raw diet and two weeks of a therapeutic diet, regular meals should always be preceded by fruit and raw salads, while coffee, black tea, alcoholic beverages, nicotine, sweets, chocolate, and greasy, fried, and baked dishes should be avoided. In the beginning, do not eat eggs, cheese, or meat. A little milk may be consumed, but in unsweetened form (sour milk, bioyogurt, yogurt, buttermilk, see pages 84-85).

The beginning of the changeover is not easy. It must be fought out. Success gradually becomes apparent to an increasing degree. It is understandable that frequent migraine attacks must be expected in the beginning, since the diet conversion has precisely the same aim as a migraine itself, that is, the elimination of undesirable substances, general discharge of the tissue, and flow of bile. As a result, fatigue, drowsiness, feelings of heaviness and dullness disappear only slowly. They disappear to the degree that purification is effected; genuine cure goes along with this.

Large amounts of urine and improved operation of the digestive organs are the first signs of success. Every small step forward is simultaneously a victory over oneself, a conquering of human weakness.

The first 2 days are usually the hardest. A great amount of fatigue follows, which usually lasts 9 to 12 days, and then, another migraine. Afterwards, a stable constitution is established. Another brief attack usually occurs in the second to third week. If this is overcome, the first goal is reached. Relapses still occur easily with a change of weather, slight deficiencies in diet, excitement before or after menstruation. A complete cure can be expected only after 6 to 12 months at the earliest. The fact that many other disorders and plagues which upset a person in addition to migraines are also discharged at the same time, is a special reward for so much courage. Thus, for example, it can happen that rheumatism, varicose veins, pains in the joints, constipation, rashes, hay fever, prolonged fatigue, etc., may also disappear, and a new emotional equilibrium can be obtained.

Scheduling of Time, Exercise—Rest, Use of Water

A well-ordered schedule must also be maintained: late nights must be avoided. Whenever possible, maintain natural sleep by going to bed early, about 7 o'clock in the evening—after a walk. If going to bed so early is not suitable—by 8 o'clock at the latest. Do not get up by the clock but when you wake up yourself, and then get up even if it is before daybreak! Morning walks and frequent walks during the day are necessary for warming up—migraine patients tend to be cold. Especially valuable is stimulation of the circulation by a warm, prolonged shower, a hot and cold shower, or dry brushing of the skin in the morning. But avoid a shock from cold water, for a migraine patient easily reacts with constriction of the blood vessels. No cold baths or showers after coming out of a warm bed; always exercise first, then follow with a warm bath or shower. If you should get cold during the day, use warm affusions on the back and neck. In the evenings, rising knee-thigh baths followed by cold affusions, or calf compresses. Include regular rest periods. Sunbaths and sauna, while valuable in themselves, should be taken only after thorough medical examination and according to exact instructions. Because, if focal infections, heart pains, and similar ills exist, the careless and exaggerated use of these baths could activate them. A migraine may be provoked by such unthinking harsh treatment.

Drugs

It is absolutely necessary to dispense with all headache remedies (even ergotamine, which regulates the tone of blood vessels), for every effect of attenuation or retardation is harmful to the improvement of the excretion process and can hinder the success of the cure or even aggravate a migraine. However, the homeopathic method of natural plant-remedy extracts as used in phytotherapy (the use of vegetable drugs in medicine), or herb tea as proffered by nature, can be of welcome assistance (see Recipe and Menu section, herb tea). The doctor must decide on the selection of homeopathic remedies.

Massage, Autogenic Training, and Exercise

Connective-tissue massage of the neck and forehead regions along nerve endings and orbital cavities has proven to be of particular value to migraine patients. Then, under the supervision of a doctor, the patient can receive *autogenic training* (self-regulation of the physical and emotional aspects of the body) for physical and spiritual relaxation. Autogenic Training is a system of self-regulation devised by Johannes Schultz (early 20th century), and is based on self-hypnosis, Yoga, and Eastern disciplines. This also includes breathing and posture exercises, general relaxation and exercises to make the spine more flexible.

A new feeling for the body must be awakened, which should include gymnastic instruction, in which tension is overcome, and a harmonious coordination of movement to bring about bodily awareness.

Treatment of Emotional Aspects

Any migraine treatment must be based on an understanding of the personality as a whole; the "language" of migraines must be understood. A migraine, or headache, as a symptom is often based on unconsciously forced suppression of developmental phases and desires. Constriction of the blood vessels is then an expression of emotional blocking and bracing, of "painful" torment and depression. The basis of the preparation for a cure of any disease is laid by the self-development and self-knowledge of the patient by an awareness of the body's interrelationships. A solution to harassing obligations, a professional or locational change, can bring ostensible help. But this help is only of value if its deeper meaning is recognized, and if the change in the external framework is not merely an effort to escape from realistic claims.

A fulfilled, healthy life is a protection against many diseases, whereas isolation and lack of goals promote illness. This applies especially to a migraine. Unconditional dedication to a task is probably the best recovery for a human soul. The call to such a task is not only a favor of fate: If he is inwardly prepared, every person can become sensitive to tasks which enrich his life and bring him fulfillment. At the same time, the longing for security, human contact, inner and external guidance and belief, basic needs of all human beings, are usually satisfied.

A talk with a clergyman, a physician, and a psychotherapist, the study of Christian and Eastern teachings of wisdom, can point the way to knowledge and healing. Meditation and Yoga are often a great help. Yoga does not only mean Hatha Yoga, but a genuine "science of liberation"–"mastery of disorder and ignorance through inner and external purity, truth, moderation, study, humility, and devotion to God," as described by the old scriptures.* In connection with this, it should be emphasized that a metabolically overloaded, exhausted, or diseased person is incapable of such brainwork. Care, control, and purification of the body are indispensable prerequisites.

What to Do in an Acute Migraine Attack

What should you do if the massive attacks, with their total force of destructive and despairing feelings, overcome you? Where can you find the strength to hold out without a pain reliever? There are a whole series of practical, valuable, and helpful measures available for this purpose. They bring relief without upsetting the healing process. Above all: Do not reach for a pain-killer right off!

If a migraine begins upon awakening, and is still rather light, try a few minutes of autogenous-training, exercise** and then go for an early walk. The attack is often overcome by relaxation followed thereafter by stimulating the circulation. If the attack is already full-blown however, then complete submission on the spot is the order of the day: bed rest, wide open windows, dim lights, limitation of food intake to sips of fruit juices and different kinds of herb tea of sour and bitter content, such as: some diluted, unsweetened lemon juice, grapefruit juice, orange juice, peppermint or anise tea lightly sweetened with honey, grape juice, carrot juice, beet juice—only natural sources of

---
*Yoga Sara Sangraha, *Vishnana Bhiksu*, Theosophical Publishing House, Adyar Madras.
**See Exercises, Page 153.

sugar. Refined sugar causes vomiting during a migraine attack. Let thin, sour apple slices dissolve in your mouth. Fat should never be touched!

Some patients can cut short the threatening attack at the start by eating a lot of food. In this way, the organism can be forced, by the increased work of digestion, to suppress its purification crisis (and uric acid metabolic products). This is no better than gulping down drugs.

Hot neck compresses—very hot and laid along the spine from the neck down to the lumbar region, with the cloth folded over eight times—can often bring amazing relief. The compresses can be repeated several times during the day. In case of abdominal cramps, apply hot abdominal compresses. Take care that hands and feet are warm. The eyes must be relaxed consciously. Small finger massages over the eyebrows, into the forehead, and over the temples, plus the warm palms of your hands on these areas often work wonders. A piece of dark cloth laid over the eyes promotes full relaxation of the eyes.

During the attack, a good recumbent position is important. The head must be comfortable. The neck must not be bent at all. It is best to use an herbal chaff or fleece cushion (or neckroll). Blood vessels leading up to the head must not be pressed and tight. The knees should also be supported somewhat by a roll. During the migraine attack, an expert massage of connective tissue (ligaments, tendons, etc.) can be of great help: the painful areas, the places where nerve endings are close to the surface on the back of the head and over the orbital cavities, are relaxed and loosened with gentle stroking. The painfully cramped muscles from the neck on down to those over the shoulders and the sternum are loosened and stretched. Additional special treatment with acupuncture and neural therapy can bring great relief, depending, of course, on the doctor's decision.

If the attack fades slowly, a prolonged mild, warm bath (of 98.6°) for 30-40 minutes is wonderfully relaxing and comforting.

The difficult hours can be overcome by using all of your strength. "He who conquers the hour, conquers the day, and he who conquers the day, conquers the year." The patient must feel that he is surrounded by calm and trust, and that friends are standing by him. He himself deserves encouragement and respect for his perseverance, and should be allowed to feel it. He has to know that perseverance will conquer the illness and overcome his dependency on pain pills. If everyone around him cooperates in the same spirit and shows the same willingness to help, such a time of struggle and self-discipline can become a milestone in the life and development of the patient.

A Few Examples

First Case: A forty-four-year-old woman goes to the doctor's office with very severe migraines that she has had for ten years. She receives injections of ergotamine preparations three to four times a week. If the injection is not given promptly in the morning, when the pressure in her head is still weak, then very severe hemicranial migraine results for as long as two to three days.

This woman's early history is typical: As a young girl, she was ill with pancreatic tuberculosis. She later had severe chronic constipation, which became even stronger with pregnancies. She leads an extremely active social life, is accustomed to aperitifs, cocktails, and smoking—more than twenty cigarettes a day (nicotine is a typical constrictive poison)—and needs coffee at least three times a day. Restlessness, haste, and inner tension have become her permanent life companions. The war years, with a series of profound changes and upsets in her life have deepened her emotionally tense condition.

In the last two years, the patient has aged drastically. She looks care-worn, emaciated, and is deteriorated in appearance. Her skin has a noticeably grey color and a loose, wrinkled, dry quality to it. She is often in a deep depression.

She comes in for clinical care. A "battle with the devil" follows: enduring the migraine without injections! The storm breaks out two to three times every second day: tormenting pain, continual vomiting of water and bile, the feeling that she is going to die.

She lies in a darkened, fully aired room. Her intestine is cleared with a camomile enema. On her whole back up to her neck, long, narrow, hot-water compresses are laid and frequently changed. When the tendency to vomit subsides, she is given diluted lemon or orange juice, tea from bitter herbs such as peppermint, anise, centaury (an herb often used as a tonic), and common Benedict, or an alkaline, noncarbonated mineral water which is administered in sips. (Among the homeopathically effective means we might note, nux vomica, gelsemia, spigelia, and bryonia.) All conversation is discontinued. Calm reigns. And thus the patient pulls through. After every migraine-treatment experience, there is an ever-stronger feeling of relief and freshness, in addition to greater fatigue and more relief of tension. The abundant flow of urine declines the third time. The interval between attacks increases to three, four, and eight days. Then there are three weeks without migraines, a good appetite, and a feeling of well-being not previously known. There is no desire for coffee, tobacco, or even alcoholic beverages now. She instinctively wants fresh fruit, green lettuce, hard whole-wheat bread that takes a long time to chew, and clabbered milk. A very light, final migraine follows after three weeks. Afterwards, there are years of complete freedom from headaches and injections.

Second Case: Mrs. M.K. had hemicranial migraines for years in weekly attacks. She was found to have a purulent gall-bladder infection. Treatment: emptying and disinfection of the intestine. Then juice fasts followed by raw-diet periods and a fat-free diet rich in raw food. After four weeks of treatment, no more migraines. Two years later: She has not had a migraine since.

Third Case: Mrs. H.S. suffered from very severe migraines and constipation: general physical and nervous exhaustion; had a tense appearance. Intestinal activity severely disturbed. Increased bile value in blood. Treatment: raw diet, rest, *autogenous training,* massage, choleretic herb extract to stem the flow of bile. After three weeks, the migraine was visibly improved and the intestine functioning normally. The patient remained free of migraines except after exceptional overindulgence and consumption of alcohol and after strong emotional excitement—when short, mild pains still occur.

Fourth Case: Miss K.J.: Migraines once a week. Severe constipation. Half-hour lunchtime during which she eats meat only, and her concerned mother gives her the same at home. The migraine began when she was twenty-two after a disappointing love affair and a change of occupation (telephone operator). Black tea and pain killers (ergotamine) help less and less. With a radical conversion of diet—two weeks of raw diet, then a vegetable diet of 60 to 70 percent raw food, and herbal baths—she is completely well. A sporadic migraine still occurs with a change in weather.

Fifth Case: Mrs. E.V.: Migraine attacks after the birth of her third child. Excited, overstimulated. High blood pressure. Much black tea, alcohol, social engagements. Chronic tonsilitis. Anemia as a result of strong menstrual bleeding due to myoma. Constipation. Gall-bladder infection. Treatment: low-fat raw diet. Three times daily, gall bladder drainage, abstinence from black tea and alcohol. Tonsilectomy. The migraine was subdued after six months. Blood pressure normal, bowel movement good. Further bleeding during menopause: Myomectomy. A few migraine attacks recur. Later, improvement and full healing without recurrence of migraines.

Sixth Case: Mrs. R.M.: Beginning at twenty-four, she lost twenty pounds and had a migraine once a week after pregnancy: severest form with rotary vertigo, lasting for three days. Irregular menstrual periods. Abuse of coffee and pain killers. Anemia. Intestinal decay, lack of hydrochloric acid. Treatment: Juice fast. Raw diet. Abstinence from drugs and coffee. Massage and administration of stomach enzymes. Massage of ligaments, tendons and other connective tissue. Learning autogenous training. Rest. The migraine disappeared and stayed away about three years. It did not appear again until her husband became ill and she took over the business. Since then, she is free of illness, except for times of special stress.

Seventh Case: Mrs. B.F. suffered from very severe migraines since youth. Daily in the morning. Two to six pills a day. Diet consists mainly of meat and white bread. Fresh food lacking. Her husband overactive, and the atmosphere was constantly tense. Increase of uric acid in the blood. Eczema on hands and neck. Cardialgia. Anemia from drug poisoning. Arthrosis of cervical vertebrae. Overweight. Depressed. Insomnia. Treatment: Conversion of diet. Abstinence from drugs. Rest. Massage. Autogenous training. After 3 weeks, the patient was free of pain. Since then, migraines occurred only in connection with nervous stress, if the patient had to keep up with the excessive pace of her husband and if her diet was deficient. At such times, she also reached for pain pills. The recurrences became less and less frequent, however, as Mrs. F. freed herself of her addiction. Her weight remains "slim." Chronic convulsive constipation is overcome by the continuing diet. The eczema healed up completely.

Migraine Prevention

Many people who are plagued with migraines genuinely would like to find the courage and strength to overcome them. Bircher-Benner said: "The road lies before you. It is up to you to travel it."

Parents who give their children an example of a harmonious and healthy family life are doing the most valuable thing to prevent migraines and many other chronic physical and emotional illnesses. This harmony also includes a good diet rich in vital materials and a regulated daily schedule.

In their weekly menus, every family should try to introduce at least one raw-food day, with only fruit, salad, fresh grain, and nuts. On the remaining days, every meal should begin with fresh fruit. Whole-wheat bread should normally be used instead of refined white bread and sweets should definitely be avoided. There should be ten minutes of exercise daily at an open window, if the outside air is pure enough. Neck exercises are especially important.* Try to avoid prolonged tension. If it occurs daily, countermeasures must be provided. When possible, there should be a longer weekend, in which quiet, harmonious, relaxing family gatherings are important. Executives and career women should do this every two or three months. Relax, and occupy yourself with your favorite pastime; seek out your hidden talents and your life will be more fulfilling. Keep your ambitions to yourself and do not transfer them to your children. Set an example of consideration and tolerance for them. As often as possible, children should be given quiet, loving attention and their childish worries should be taken seriously. A harmonious development is more important than a perfect notebook in

---

*See Neck Exercises, Page 153.

school and a brilliant career. Most important, a relationship to nature and respect for living things should be maintained. When material things are valued more than peace of mind, it is time to evaluate your life, and the basic cause of countless diseases—such as migraine—can be overcome. The whole person is cured—he develops and fulfills his life meaningfully.

How Bircher-Benner Describes the Relationship Between the Metabolic State and Migraines

The excellent description by Bircher-Benner of the relationship between the metabolic condition and symptoms of illness, although done some years ago, is still very contemporary and its truth has been confirmed by very recent research on a large number of other metabolic developments. (Naturally, some updating is necessary to include the latest findings of physiological chemistry, since uric acid is not the only cause of the reactions described below.) From: *Nutritional Illnesses,* first part by Dr. M. Bircher-Benner (Wendepunkt Publishing Co., Zurich, 1927), pp. 130-137:

> Dr. Haig controlled the excretion of uric acid in the urine from hour to hour, from day to day, from season to season; he simultaneously determined the uric acid content of the blood, followed the phenomena detected in the circulation of the blood, and the objective and subjective syndrome. Comparing one series of operations with another, he came to the conclusion that his migraine was caused by the flooding of his blood with uric acid. He supplied himself with a certain amount of uric acid, either in his diet or as a chemical substance, observed its course through his blood and its excretion in his urine, and experienced a headache again. He learned to lower the supply and production of uric acid in his body to a minimum and remarked that the headaches disappeared noticeably for an arbitrarily long time. Without exception, his blood was overloaded with uric acid when he had a headache and, without exception, the headache occurred when he intentionally overloaded his blood with uric acid. A headache never occurs without excessive amounts of uric acid in the blood, whether from the diet or elsewhere.

But the amount of uric acid in the blood also depends, as Haig soon recognized, on whether the blood contains enough solvent, certain alkalies (bases). If a lot of uric acid is dissolved in the blood and is removed from it by consuming acids which require the solvent (the base) of the blood for themselves, the uric acid is then thrown out of the blood into the tissue, especially into the joints, periostea, cartilage, and connective tissue. The blood then becomes free of uric acid, but the tissue becomes laden with it and irritating symptoms appear. The headache attack also disappears in this way, but the uric acid causing it has by no means been excreted from the body. It remains in the tissue. It can remain there and new amounts of uric acid can be added, day by day, so that a considerable store of uric acid gradually forms in the tissues mentioned. This will most certainly be the case if daily nourishment supplies excess acidity instead of excess alkalinity (any diet that is rich in protein will do this, especially a diet that has an abundant amount of meat). With migraine patients, however, an internal situation always occurs in which the uric-acid load of the blood increases into a wave of headaches. If the blood has already accumulated a store of uric acid, the attacks then occur when uric-acid free food is eaten, since the uric acid in the tissues breaks through from time to time and flows back into the blood.

Uric acid in the blood means excretion of uric acid by the kidneys. Thus excretion, and, therefore, relief to the body, also depend on a sufficient amount of solvent (base) in the blood. If a lot of uric acid is in the urine, then there is little in the blood. But this does not prove that no uric acid is being formed. As a rule, this proves that the solvent is consumed by other acids, whereas the uric acid continually being formed and supplied is stored in the tissues and accumulates there. Preceding the headache is a stage in which the sick person feels especially well and fresh. In the course of this stage, he excretes very bright urine containing very little uric acid, and his blood is exceptionally low in uric acid. The uric acid coming from the food, is retained in the tissues only suddenly to break through later into the blood like a hurricane, causing a headache attack. Many sick people know this stage and know that suffering will soon recur, while others regularly misunderstand their feeling of well-being and believe an improvement is now really occurring. They express their joyful hopes to friends or to their doctor. A few hours later, their little ship of hope lies shattered on a rock. This peculiar phenomenon also occurs in many other illnesses in which uric acid is the cause. Even many years ago, a warning call arose inside me if a sick person enthusiastically boasted of his feeling of well-being and improvement. Experience had taught me that the following day would bring a worse recurrence.

"Exulting to the high heavens leads to deathly grief" can also be said of uric acid. Similar phenomena occur in many women before menstruation, but it is certainly well known that the migraine attacks occur particularly toward the time of the period, and Haig has shown that uric acid upheavals always take place around that time. Since the formation of uric acid and its movement through the blood is internally related to the metabolic processes as a whole, a striking periodicity is apparent many times in the effects of uric acid, which develops synchronously with the periodicity of the metabolism. Haig, by following these periodic occurrences daily and comparing them with each other, discovered a daily period and an annual period in the effects of uric acid. First, this is what he says about the daily period:

Sir W. Roberts, the English metabolic researcher, had pointed out that in our organism a daily fluctuation between excess acidity and alkalinity takes place. The acids control the metabolic processes from 11 A.M. on into the night and reach their peak about 11 P.M. The alkalies or bases, on the other hand, assume control after midnight, by 4 A.M. at the latest, and maintain control until about 11 A.M. with their peak about 9 A.M. Roberts compared this fluctuation with the tides of the sea and called the time of alkaline control the alkaline flow. Corresponding to this alteration between acidic and alkaline control, Haig now discovered the course of uric acid through the blood. During the period of acidic control, the blood contains little uric acid, just as the urine, which is bright and copious upon excretion; the hampering effects of uric acid on the circulation of the blood in the capillaries, about which we will soon have more to say, are absent, so that circulation and perfusion of tissue develop favorably. During this period, the uric acid being formed and supplied in food is more or less retained in organs and tissues. Things proceed inversely during the alkaline flow. With the predominance of bases, the blood becomes more and more laden with uric acid and its excretion by the kidneys increases. In the course of this, the urine becomes dark and decreases in volume. Of course, uric acid also affects circulation and capillaries. The flow of the laden blood in the capillaries slows down, the perfusion of tissue becomes more sluggish, and finally oxygen begins to decrease and carbon dioxide accumulates, resulting ultimately in carbon dioxide poisoning. The strength of these disturbances, according to Haig, depends primarily on excess uric acidity in the metabolism.

During the predominance of acidity, which recurs every day at the same time, the uric acid accordingly becomes congested in the tissues, the blood is thus freed from it, circulation in the capillaries speeds up, and the diluted urine which is low in uric acid flows out copiously through the kidneys, which makes the person feel comfortable, well, healthy, strong, and energetic. At the time of alkaline flow, conditions are reversed: the congested uric acid flows back into the blood, and appears in large amounts in the now dark and meager amount of urine. The greater the amount of uric acid, the more sensitive the disturbance of capillary circulation becomes, and through it, damage to the exchange of gases. The feeling of well being worsens to the same degree. Discomfort, lassitude, heaviness in limbs and head, aversion, and bad humor set in. These are symptoms of the effect of uric acid, which in many people, from day to day, become even stronger on waking up in the morning after a deep sleep. In many people, these symptoms disappear after getting up and after vigorous muscular exercise, as the latter can restore capillary circulation in light cases. Others use a cold shower or a cold bath, whose refreshing effect they cannot praise highly enough. This kind of refreshment, however, as Haig showed, is expensive, since, in the course of this, the uric acid dissolved in the blood and destined for excretion, is simply thrown back into the tissue, from whence it flows back into the blood at the next opportunity or is used to increase the store of uric acid, which, as we will see, then prepares the way for rheumatism, arthritis, and other diseases in later life. Pure coffee, black tea, chocolate, and cocoa work in a very similar way. Today these drinks seem to be indispensable breakfast drinks for so many people. Their content of xanthine substances—elements of uric acid—makes it possible for them to take the solvent out of the blood, after which the uric acid clears from the blood and is again thrown back into the tissues. It is therefore understandable that the love for these drinks increases to the extent that the amount of uric acid, which is ready for the alkaline flow, increases in the body. But this amount of uric acid also increases directly through these drinks, whose xanthine is converted into uric acid in the metabolism. Without suspecting it, the devil in this instance is driven away by Beelzebub.

The uric acid effect of the alkaline flow, with abundant uric acid production, can become so strong that the sleeper wakes up every morning with limbs as heavy as lead or with headaches.

Many can hardly move on rising, and there are even some among the "nervous," as well as among the "weak," who do not leave their beds before 11 A.M. and are fully convinced that their health can no longer stand an early rising at all. Contributing to this conviction are, particularly, heart pains, which are associated with circulatory disturbances in high degrees of this morning uric acid and carbon-dioxide poisoning. These circulatory disturbances do not go away again until the blood is cleared of uric acid by the rise of acidity. In a definite slant, all such people slowly slide to their downfall. Apart from the constant accumulation of the store of uric acid, they suffer from a progressive sensitive weakening of the most fragile and most important organs of the body as a result of the period of lack of oxygen and of carbon-dioxide poisoning which increases every few hours, daily. These fragile organs include, in particular, the brain, the spinal cord, and the sympathetic nervous system.

The number of people, some even very young, who have to bear such morning upsets is very large. As a rule, neither they themselves nor their doctors know anything about the causative relationships mentioned here and discovered by Alexander Haig. Treatment corresponds to this lack of knowledge. In the case of weak people, it is almost always decided that they just simply cannot stand to get up early. They should therefore not get out of bed before 10 or 11 A.M. Thus they lie in bed every fine morning of their lives, their organs decaying in carbon-dioxide poisoning and their willpower, so necessary for organizing their lives, slowly dies. After a few years, severe illnesses set in, but the lack of knowledge of relationships is also what makes this possible. With regard to diet, they behave exactly as Haig did before he cured himself of his despair: they try to strengthen these "powerless" systems with "powerful" nourishment—as much meat, eggs, meat extract, and bouillon as possible—they drink coffee, tea, to "wake up." If heart pains occur, they obtain caffeine, a concentrated xanthine-uric acid preparation. All these measures, however, only increase the supply of uric acid to the body, as the excretion of uric acid becomes more and more possible; the excess acidity of foods rich in protein cause the supply of uric acid to become larger and larger.

And yet there is a very simple method of transforming the entire condition completely within a short time. But no one thinks of this way, unless the one in ten thousand who is in deepest despair. This remedy is: stop eating meat, eggs, coffee, tea, and bouillon, and substitute a diet that is low in uric acid, high in bases and vitamins, with fresh fruit, fruitlike vegetables, salads, raw vegetables, potatoes, and correctly cooked vegetables. In addition to this, get lots of exercise in the early morning's fresh air, take walks, and when possible, a sunbath. Who once understands these relationships, asks himself: But why are people so blind that they cannot see this? The explanation for this behavior lies, as we will also see, in the effects of uric acid itself.

The processes of daily periodicity described above, and precisely expressed in the acidic-and-alkaline flow theory of Sir W. Roberts, furnish us with very unexpected conclusions concerning the effects of uric acid on our subjective feeling of well-being. We do not sense whether or not we are consuming little or much uric acid in food, nor whether little or much uric acid is present in our body. We feel only that little or much uric acid is present in our blood. As soon as the uric-acid content of the blood exceeds a certain amount, which is probably different for every individual, we become uncomfortable. The result of hampered circulation and carbon dioxide poisoning is weakness, stiffness in the limbs, a heavy head and in many people, a headache itself. We will soon see that a series of diseased conditions develop in connection with prolonged overloading of the blood with uric acid.

We also do not sense whether or not we are excreting uric acid supplied and produced during the day, or whether we are accumulating a portion of it, often a very considerable portion in the tissues. We can accumulate it for years, but until arthritis finally breaks out, we do not notice it. We completely misinterpret the opportune warning signals whose diversity we will also soon learn to recognize, and consider them "cold illnesses" or "nervous conditions" and combat them with remedies which only aggravate their causative condition.

We only sense an increased, pleasant feeling when the blood is free of uric acid and a heavy, hampered, depressed, and unpleasant feeling when the blood is laden with uric acid. The first condition suits us, the second does not. We do not want to have any uric acid in our blood. Our behavior is accordingly directed and explained.

Freeing the blood from uric acid can be accomplished in two different, diametrically opposed ways. The first way is to select a diet that is relatively free of uric acid; the second way is to clear the blood of uric acid by acids, in which case the uric acid is driven into the tissue of our bodies and stored.

III. Menus

Fasting is a special type of body cleansing and water reduction, regeneration, and recuperation, in migraine patients signifying a process which should occur at the beginning of the general changeover. The degree and length of time of the fast are to be strictly determined according to the orders of the doctor.

Fasts

Tea Fasts and Juice Fasts

Distinguish between tea fasts and juice fasts. Tea fasts are used when nausea makes it impossible to accept nourishment, as in the condition of acute migraines.

Administer camomile tea in sips with a few drops of unsweetened lemon juice, a spoonful at a time. In place of camomile tea, peppermint tea, bitter tea, tea for relieving gas, balm-mint tea, or verbena tea can also be used. In place of tea, occasionally let very thin slices of apples dissolve in your mouth or chew a peppermint leaf.

When the migraine has passed its climax and vomiting subsides, a juice fast follows, consisting of 5-7 ounces of fruit or vegetable juice. Use fresh fruit juices depending on the season. Drink one spoonful at a time as in tea fasts, if the acute migraine condition has already faded and thirst still prevails. Especially recommended are grapes (unsprayed only), citrus fruit (not too sour), especially grapefruit and mandarin oranges, all berries, and apples.

Amount: 21-35 ounces per day, alternating or diluted with tea or uncarbonated mineral water. In place of fruit juices, fresh vegetable juices can be used: carrot, beet, and raw potato juice, as a small admixture. The amount should be distributed 4-5 times daily. In case of thirst, drink herb tea in swallows, made from peppermint, wormwood, or centaury, and possibly also boiled vegetable broth, free of fat and salt.

It is important to have good bowel evacuation. If necessary, take an enema in the morning and evening, and 1-2 tablespoons ground soaked flax-seed or sessile leaves or fleawort (also called psyllium) per day (soaked beforehand for one hour in one glass of water or apple juice).

A fresh juice fast can be carried on for as long as several days, or even up to two to three weeks, according to a doctor's prescription. Medical supervision during the fast and during the subsequent period of restructuring is important. Professional work and great physical and emotional tension are undesirable at this time. If only a mild effect of fasting is desired for prevention of migraines, general detoxification, drainage and rejuvenation, a strict fruit-juice day can be introduced once a week. In the case of female migraine patients, the juice day is especially important before menstruation. With longer fasts, full bed rest is necessary during the first to tenth days of fasting, otherwise the optimum effect is lost since it is destroyed by fatigue, and good appetite and correct relaxation are not attained. Do not be discouraged by reactions such as headaches, nausea, pains in the limbs, feelings of weakness (especially at noon). In juice fasts, these are indications that the body is beginning the work of detoxification. Thus, such days fulfill their purpose. However, report your observations to your doctor. A strong flow of urine should be regarded as a good sign on juice days.

Full Juice Fast (Liquid Diet)

Morning: 7 oz. fruit juice
5 oz. skim milk or yogurt
1 cup rose hip tea or other kind of tea

Noon: 7 oz. fruit juice
5 oz. almond milk or yogurt
5 oz. vegetable juice

Evening: Same as morning

A high-quality, relatively nutritious, but very light diet is supplied here. This form of diet can be continued for a week or longer without reducing full daily activity. Full juice periods are suitable at the beginning of conversion treatments for migraine patients and also in cases of the body's great impoverishment in life-supporting substances, as is usually the case with migraines.

Fruit juice can first be mixed with 1/3 flaxseed (or linseed), barley or rice water. In dehydration cures, urination and weight must be watched; if necessary, a diuretic tea such as rose hip can be taken.

Fruit Fast Day

Whole-fruit fasts can replace juice fasts if, for example, metabolic improvement and intestinal stimulation through the cellulose (that is in the fruit pulp) are desired. There is a greater feeling of satiation and a fruit fast can, therefore, be carried on for a whole day without complete rest, and for even longer periods. However, the effect of the juice fast is more intensive. A fruit fast is advisable in the case of migraine patients suffering from intestinal sluggishness.

Daily Menu

Seven to eleven ounces of organic, well-washed, fresh, completely ripe, unsweetened fruit, three times daily, berries, citrus fruit (oranges, tangerines, grapefruits, mandarin oranges), grapes, figs, melons, Japanese persimmons. If available, papayas, fresh pineapples, fresh young coconuts (milk and white flesh), avocados, mangoes, ripe bananas, and pomegranates are also very valuable. Sprayed fruit must be peeled.

If diarrhea occurs, a fruit day of grated apples only is advised.

Special Forms of Fruit Fasts

Apple day: 5-6 times daily, 1 large apple finely grated if migraines with acute gastroenteritis and diarrhea occur.

Strawberry day: 3-4 times daily, 7-9 oz. very ripe, unsweetened strawberries. High in Vitamin C content, nourishing, and thirst quenching. It maintains healthy intestinal flora. The strawberry season should be taken advantage of.

Blueberry day: 3-4 times daily, 7-9 oz. blueberries, slightly constipating and disinfecting to the intestine.

Blackberry day: 3 times daily, 7-11 oz. completely ripe blackberries. Especially rich in natural sugar and Vitamin C. Nourishing and easily digestible. (Has the effect of soothing and reducing swelling in the throat and vocal chords.)

Currant day: 3 times daily, 7-9 oz. currants (2/3 red and white, 1/3 black). Especially refreshing and thirst-quenching in cases of migraines with liver disorders. Rich in Vitamin C.

Japanese Persimmon day: 4 times daily, 2 small or 1 large Japanese persimmons. Very nourishing and rich in Vitamins B and C.

Grape day: (famous old grape cure) 4-5 times daily, 1-2 lbs. sun-ripened grapes, unsprayed, if possible. Wash well (rinse briefly in hot water) and eat the fruit whole. Although poor in vitamins, grapes are especially nourishing because of their high glucose content, for liver protection, drainage, and intestinal stimulation (from the seeds). Grape cures can be taken for a week in autumn.

Papaya day: 3 times daily, 1/2 large papaya with lemon juice. It promotes stomach digestion through the papain found in papayas. Rich in fructose and Vitamins B and C.

Raw Food

Fresh raw-food nutrition is the basis of dietetic alteration, weight reduction, bodily regeneration, and is the beginning of dietetic therapy for migraine patients. A harmonious distribution of tuberous, root, and leafy raw vegetables must be provided, always fresh and fully ripe.

Menus for the Raw-Food Day:

Morning: Bircher Muesli with fruit or berries and whole-grain flakes
1 tbsp. sprouted wheat (must be well chewed), wheat germ, nuts, or presoaked sunflower seeds.
dried fruit
1 glass almond milk, certified, sour, or buttermilk
1 cup rose hip, fennel, or lime-blossom tea with lemon juice and honey (instead of sugar).

Noon: Generous fruit platter
nuts, raisins, dates, or dried banana
raw vegetables as Boston lettuce, celery root, tomatoes, or, cucumbers, carrots, watercress
or, sauerkraut, beets, fennel
as supplement, 1 or 2 potatoes cooked in their jackets
or, fresh vegetable broth, 1 glass certified milk (unpasteurized), sour, almond, soy bean, or buttermilk.

52 Nutrition Plan for Headache and Migraine Patients

Evening: Bircher Muesli prepared in different ways, depending on the season, that is, a variety of fruit and nuts, fruit pastes
or, 4 dried figs, cut up and soaked in apple juice, mixed with 1-1/3 cups of sour milk or yogurt,
or, raw whole-grain Muesli sweetened with grape or pear juice, mixed with frothily beaten bananas and lemon or orange juice
as dressing, light cream or certified milk
1 cup herb tea sweetened with honey (instead of sugar).

A Week's Raw-Food Diet Menus According to the Season

Planning menus is, of course, determined by what is available during different seasons. (This is a list of a week's seasonal raw foods possible during each season of the year.)

a) Spring

    1st day: fruit-nuts (also dried fruit)-radishes-fennel-Boston lettuce
    2nd day: fruit-nuts-celery root-tomatoes-watercress
    3rd day: fruit-nuts-carrots-Belgian endives-Boston lettuce
    4th day: fruit-nuts-turnips-Romaine lettuce-watercress
    5th day: fruit-nuts-beets-dandelion-Boston lettuce
    6th day: fruit-nuts-cauliflower-spinach-watercress
    7th day: fruit-nuts-kohlrabi-tomatoes-Boston lettuce

b) Summer

    1st day: fruit-nuts-radish-tomatoes-Boston lettuce
    2nd day: fruit-nuts-carrots-zucchini-Boston lettuce
    3rd day: fruit-nuts-kohlrabi-watercress-Boston lettuce
    4th day: fruit-nuts-cauliflower-radish-Boston lettuce
    5th day: fruit-nuts-celery-Romaine lettuce-Boston lettuce
    6th day: fruit-nuts-tomatoes stuffed with cauliflower-Boston lettuce
    7th day: fruit-nuts-carrots-cucumbers-Boston lettuce

c) Autumn

    1st day: fruit-nuts-celery root-tomatoes-endive
    2nd day: fruit-nuts-beets-bell peppers-Boston lettuce
    3rd day: fruit-nuts-viper's grass-spinach-Boston lettuce
    4th day: fruit-carrots-zucchini-watercress-lettuce
    5th day: fruit-nuts-cauliflower-lettuce-endive
    6th day: fruit-nuts-turnips-tomatoes-Boston lettuce
    7th day: fruit-nuts-celery-cucumbers-Boston lettuce

d) Winter

    1st day: fruit-nuts-viper's grass-red cabbage-endive
    2nd day: fruit-nuts-celery-red chicorino-Boston lettuce
    3rd day: fruit-nuts-carrots-bell peppers-Boston lettuce
    4th day: fruit-nuts-beets-sauerkraut-endive
    5th day: fruit-nuts-cauliflower-spinach-lettuce
    6th day: fruit-nuts-tomatoes-Belgian endives-Boston lettuce
    7th day: fruit-nuts-celery roots-savoy cabbage-endive

Single Raw-Food Diet

A single-food diet means eating only *one* kind of food at each meal. This is a transition from fasting and a raw diet to a prolonged diet and provides a considerably smaller load for the digestive organs and liver than a mixed menu. It consists of three meals.

Morning: Apples (eaten slowly and chewed well) as much as you want, or another kind of fruit, as, grapes, grapefruit, berries, cherries, or even tomatoes, etc.

Noon: Millet puree, or steamed potatoes, or a wheat dish, or selected steamed vegetables; the amount depends on your appetite. Eat slowly.

Evening: As at noon, but chew vegetables well; if potatoes were eaten at noon, or vice versa, then substitute crispbread.

10 A.M. and 4 P.M.   Juices or herb tea in small sips as described in juice and tea-fast day.

The single-food day should be carried out more or less strictly. The gastric juices of the stomach are relieved through the simplification of the demands upon them, and nausea subsides. Should severe vomiting and heartburn occur, take kaolin with some bitter tea between meals, and 1 tbsp. fresh potato juice 1-2 times daily. This single-food day is also beneficial after severe migraine attacks.

Therapeutic Diet for Migraine Patients: Menus for Prolonged Periods

Guidelines: Low-fat to nonfat diet, depending on the doctor's prescription. Avoid fried and irritating foods, sharp spices, vegetables causing gas, and sweets. Chew well, eat slowly, rest after meals, keep warm. Thus, correct care of the stomach, intestine, and liver is assured.

Low-Fat Diet (as a prolonged diet for migraine patients):

Morning: 4 oz. portion of Bircher Muesli with yogurt
1 tsp. pine kernels or groundnuts
whole-wheat bread or crispbread with 1/3 tbsp. butter or diet margarine, honey, herb tea without sugar.

Noon: Fruit
raw vegetables with cottage cheese or yogurt dressing, or with a very little oil and plenty of fresh herbs
carrots, tomatoes, celery root, all green lettuces, beets, zucchini, spinach, and radish are suitable. (Cabbages and viper's grass are not used, as they are somewhat gas-producing.)

Follow with either soup (uncreamed) made with very little butter (e.g., tomato or rolled-oat soup), or a steamed vegetable, with some fresh butter added before serving (onions pressed as juice). Carrots, fennel, celery, Romaine lettuce, zucchini, tomatoes, leeks, and spinach are especially appropriate as cooked vegetables.

As a supplement, use parsley potatoes, cereal mash, or noodles made of whole wheat, steamed without fat, and served with some fresh butter.

Fat cheese must not be used at the beginning. On the other hand, cottage cheese and low-fat soft cheese with herbs as a supplement to whole-wheat bread and potatoes, or as a dessert with fruit, are valuable complements.

Some dessert suggestions: applesauce, fruit gelatin (prepared with agar-agar or pectin), junket made from skim milk with berries, fruit salad, bananas, and apples beaten up and mixed together, and farina are also suitable. Use honey or concentrated pear juice for sweetening.

Evening: As in the morning
or, whole-wheat noodles, whole-grain rice, with tomato sauce
or, whole grits or rolled oats soup
or, cereal mash cooked with skim milk, stewed fruit
or, whole-wheat bread sandwiches (no butter) with cottage cheese and herbs, tomatoes, watercress, radish, cucumber slices, or shredded carrots.

Nonfat Diet (for migraine, liver, and gall-bladder patients):

Morning: Grated apple with some lemon juice and honey or concentrated pear juice. Whole-wheat bread or crispbread with honey
or, Bircher Muesli No. 1
or, whole-grain flakes with fruit and skim milk

or, junket made with skim milk, or buttermilk with finely cut up pitted fruit
whole-wheat bread, honey.

Noon: Fruit.

Raw vegetables can be tastefully prepared without cream and oil using powdered skim milk, which makes an excellent cream sauce when mixed with a little water. Season it with lemon juice, chopped herbs, onions, or pressed garlic or with finely grated horse radish.

Vegetable broth can also be appetizingly prepared without fat and using some sea salt and chopped parsley. Baked potatoes taste great with stewed tomatoes. Mashed potatoes can be frothily beaten with skim milk, and frothy whipped potatoes can be made by pressing potatoes through a coarse sieve. A pleasant-tasting, nourishing potato soup can also be prepared without butter by using a strong vegetable broth with marjoram, thyme, and sea salt.

Whole grain dishes need no fat to develop their delicious individual taste. In place of butter, use a seasoned tomato sauce made in a blender from fully ripe, fresh tomatoes, without cooking, but slightly warmed (Recipe No. 179).

Any fruit dish can be used as dessert, prepared without cream and fat, as for example, custards made from low fat cottage cheese with fruit juice and bananas or fruit concentrate as sweetening, or cereal mash cooked in skim milk.

Evening: Grapefruit or cold fruit soup
whole-wheat bread with honey
oat soup, without fat
grape juice or buttermilk or herb tea
or, grated apples, sliced bananas, lemon juice, corn flakes, skim or buttermilk, crispbread, tomatos, radishes, cucumber slices, apple juice or herb tea

or, 1 tomato, a few tender leaves of lettuce, chives, rice soup cooked without fat, or whole semolina cooked with skim milk. Stewed apricots without sugar.

Drink a small cup of bitter tea or some turnip juice a half hour before every meal. In the afternoon, 1 cup peppermint tea, if desired.

Diet to Prevent Constipation

As a rule, chronic constipation occurs with headaches and migraines.

Morning: Seed Muesli or Bircher Muesli with ground linseed, or whole-wheat Muesli
or, ground-wheat mash, milk, or sour milk, yogurt, kefir, buttermilk
or, fresh whole-grain flakes, fruit, sour milk or yogurt, whole-wheat bread, butter, honey
certified milk or sour milk or peppermint tea.

Noon: Berries, oranges, tangerines, or pitted fruit
raw vegetables, whole or cut into large pieces
raw health-food-store sauerkraut with some oil and yogurt
mashed potatoes, steamed zucchini, or potatoes cooked in their jackets, stuffed with peas and carrots
rhubarb sauce on toasted whole wheat bread, red currant sauce.

Evening: Bircher Muesli
or, cottage cheese and linseed oil dish as recommended by Dr. Budwig
or, whole-wheat bread, cottage cheese with horseradish, tomatoes, lettuce
or, vegetable soup
or, 4 dried figs, cut up and soaked in apple juice, as a supplement in 1 cup of sour milk or yogurt
or, raw or cooked prunes
corn on the cob with butter, herb tea.

Diet to Prevent Diarrhea

Constipation over a long period of time, accompanied by a lack of digestive juices can turn into chronic colitis with diarrhea. Acute diarrhea can also cause headaches.

Avoid grapes, citrus fruit, rhubarb, pitted fruit, fresh whole wheat bread, and sugar. Grated apples, strawberries, stewed blueberries without sugar, bananas, rice, potatoes, cottage cheese, camomile tea, soups made of cooked and strained whole meal of oats, barley, rice have a beneficial effect. Prepare all flour soups without fat and onions. Instead of raw food, first drink the juice of carrots, beets, and cabbages (does not cause gas as a juice), or potatoes. Light crispbread or Ryvita, etc.

With heavy diarrhea, start with a 1 day tea-juice fast, and bed rest. Then 1 apple day: 4-8 times a day, 1 freshly grated apple without sugar. Following the apple day and until the diarrhea disappears:

Morning: Apple muesli with crispbread, rusk, and cottage cheese, blueberry tea, or buttermilk.

Noon: Grated apples without sugar
raw vegetables with 1/3 rice water
after 3 days, finely grated carrots or beets without oil
oatmeal gruel
dry rice or potatoes with cottage cheese,
steamed tomatoes, or whole-wheat noodles with tomato sauce
applesauce.

Evening: Apple or banana, blueberry tea, whole-wheat rusk, soup or puree made from cooked, strained ground wheat or other rolled grains supplemented with crispbread, or semolina puree in milk cooked with applesauce, lightly sweetened.

Between meals: Camomile or blueberry tea in small sips, or grated apples without sugar.

Vegetable Diet (in case of allergies with migraines)

Headaches and migraines are often symptoms of allergic disorders. Therefore, in many cases a vegetable diet without animal protein is important in the beginning.

Morning: Muesli with almond puree or sesame seed and soybean
fruit according to season
whole-wheat bread, nut butter, herb tea.

Noon: Fruit
raw vegetables: beets, cucumbers, loose-leaved lettuce
cooked dishes: vegetable broth with small grits
brussel sprouts
mashed potatoes (with vegetable broth and nut butter).

Evening: As in morning.

Morning: Or, as above.

Noon: 1/2 grapefruit
raw vegetables: carrots, sauerkraut, Boston lettuce
cooked dishes: soybean soup, beets, caraway seed potatoes.

Evening: Muesli
fruit, nuts, whole-wheat bread, rose-hip preserves or marmelade
herb tea.

Morning: Or, as above.

Noon: Fruit
raw vegetables: Belgian endives with diced tomatoes and lettuce
cooked dishes: chervil soup, spinach, noodles.

Evening: Fruit
whole-grain bread with ground nuts or almond milk
fruit juice
herb tea.

Morning: Or, as above.

Noon: Fruit
raw vegetables: celery, zucchini, watercress
cooked dishes: steamed tomatoes, rice creole, orange marmelade.

Evening: Muesli
fruit
bread and nut butter
herb tea.

Salt-free Diet (for headache patients with kidney diseases who need to rid their bodies of excess fluid):

Morning: Muesli or fruit or fruit juice
whole-wheat bread (salt free)
sweet butter or nut butter (salt free)
rose-hip or other herb tea
nuts, ground or whole.

Noon: Fruit, dried fruit
raw vegetables: carrots, dandelion, head lettuce (Boston)
cooked dishes: salt-free vegetable broth with croutons
viper's grass with nut-butter sauce
tomato, potatoes.

Evening: Muesli or fruit salad or 1/2 grapefruit
soup and whole-wheat bread or baked potatoes with herb nut-butter and salad.

Morning & As above.
Evening:

Noon: Fruit
raw vegetables: beets, leeks, sauerkraut
cooked dishes: tomatoes stuffed with rice
lemon cream.

Morning & Evening:	As above.
Noon:	Fruit, dried fruit raw vegetables: radish, zucchini, head (Boston) lettuce cooked dishes: barley soup, steamed cabbage, caraway seed potatoes.
Morning & Evening:	As above.
Noon:	Fruit raw vegetables: viper's grass, tomatoes, endive cooked vegetables: spinach, cut corn, gratinee apple custard.

IV. Recipes

Bircher Muesli

1. Apple Muesli with Yogurt (1 portion)

Apple Muesli, as it was first introduced by Dr. Bircher-Benner, has remained the proven best diet dish according to our long years of experience.

As a rule, however, we replace the sweetened condensed milk originally added—especially for liver and gall bladder patients and also for migraine patients—with yogurt and honey or fruit concentrate as natural sweeteners. Refined sugar is avoided in this way. Yogurt is more easily assimilated, it aids digestion, and it is less filling.

In principle, tart, white-fleshed, juicy apples are the best, for example, Pippins, Gravensteins, Cortlands, McIntosh, Greenings, Northern Spys, Jonathans, Winesaps, and Wellingtons. If late in the season, some mealy or bland apples have to be used, their flavor can be improved by adding some freshly grated orange or lemon peel—organically grown, of course—possibly also by adding some orange juice immediately before serving and some rose-hip mash.

Depending on one's appetite, the portion can also be reduced by half.

> 1/2 oz. rolled oats (1 tbsp.)
> 3 tbsp. water
> 3 tbsp. yogurt or sour milk
> 1 tsp. lemon juice
> 1/2-1 tbsp. honey (or fruit concentrate)
> 5-7 oz. apples
> 1/2 tbsp. ground hazelnuts or almonds

Presoak oats for 12 hours in water (or use instant rolled oats if necessary). Beat yogurt, lemon juice and honey into a smooth sauce. Wash and dry apple with a clean cloth. Remove stem and core. Grate on the Bircher grater* directly into the sauce to prevent it from turning brown. (The grating should take place shortly before serving.) Sprinkle nuts over the prepared dish and use.

Wheat, rice, barley, rye, millet, buckwheat, or soybean flakes can also be used, as well as cereal grains ground in health food stores, soaked the evening before, perhaps also mixed with rolled oats (or other sources of concentrated Vitamin B). If you have a mill, freshly ground meals are best.

2. Muesli with Berries or Pitted Fruit (1 portion)

Especially high in Vitamin C.

> 5 oz. strawberries, raspberries, blueberries, currants, or blackberries
> or, 4 oz. plums, peaches, or apricots

Mash berries with a fork or a wooden pestle. Remove the pits and work through a food mill or cut up with a knife. Prepare sauce as in apple Muesli.

---

*Grater is obtainable at health-food stores.

3. Muesli with Mixed Fruit (1 portion)

Use any combination of the following fruits:

Strawberries and raspberries, or
Strawberries, raspberries, and currants, or
Strawberries and apples, or
Blackberries and apples, or
Apples with thin orange and tangerine slices, or
Apples and bananas, or
Plums and peaches or apricots, etc.

Prepare sauce as in apple Muesli.

4. Muesli with Dried Fruit (1 portion)

If circumstances require Muesli to be made with dried fruit (apples, apricots, prunes), prepare it as follows:

4 oz. dried fruit

Wash; soak in cold water for 12 hours, work through the food mill or cut up into small pieces. Blend the pulp of the fruit with the basic sauce as in apple Muesli and also use the water in which it was soaked.

Obtain good quality dried fruit without preservatives and bleaches, otherwise undesirable gastrointestinal disorders may occur.

This Muesli is especially stimulating to the intestine.

5. Raw Banana/Grain Puree (1 portion)

2 tbsp. ground grain
1/2 banana
1 tsp. honey
Lemon to taste

Soak grain 12 hours, put into blender. Mash banana and honey with a fork. Add to grain. Add lemon and serve immediately.

6. Muesli without Animal Protein (1 portion)

A vegetable dish.

    1/2 oz. rolled oats
3 tbsp. water
1 tbsp. lemon juice
1 tbsp. almond puree
1 tbsp. honey or fruit concentrate
5-7 oz. apples or berries

Soak oats for 12 hours in water. Beat lemon juice, puree, sweetener into a smooth sauce. Wash and dry fruit with a clean cloth. Remove stem and core. Grate apples on the Bircher Grater directly into the sauce.

In place of rolled oats, ground wheat, or 5-grain grind with or without linseed (also soaked for 12 hours) can be used. Instead of almond puree, ground hazelnuts or sesame seed.

7. Seed Muesli (for 1 portion)

Especially good for teeth and intestines.
On the evening before preparing, soak:

    1 tbsp. sweet dried fruit (dates, figs, raisins)
Water or apple juice
1 tbsp. whole-wheat grains or 5-grain grind
1 tbsp. sunflower seeds
2 tbsp. fresh grain flakes (cold-pressed flakes if possible)
1 tbsp. wheat germ, freshly sprouted.
1-2 tsp. walnut halves or pine kernels, ground hazelnuts or sesame seed.
Possibly some grated lemon peel (unsprayed only)

Cut dried fruit into small pieces, soak in water or apple juice. Soak whole grains 24 hours, meal only 2 hours or overnight. The water should only just cover the fruit. In the morning, add the fresh grain flakes, the wheat germ, nuts, and lemon peel.

The prepared seed Muesli should be only slightly moist, so that it stimulates good chewing. A coarsely grated apple and yogurt or sour milk can also be added before serving.

8. Maximum Mixture (1 portion)

- 2 oz. cream cheese or cottage cheese
- 8 tbsp. sour milk, yogurt, or certified milk
- 1 tsp. wheat germ oil or linseed oil
- 1 tsp. honey or pear juice
- 1 tbsp. fresh rolled grain (oats, wheat, millet, soybean, or a mixture of flakes)

Mix together cheeses, milk, wheat-germ oil, sweetener, and grain.

Or choose other supplements:
- 1 tsp. ground linseed
- 1 tsp. sunflower seeds
- 1 tbsp. ground wheat
- 1 tsp. grapes or raisins
- 1 tsp. pine nuts or walnuts or almonds
- Grated lemon peel (unsprayed only), if desired

Soak seeds and wheat in apple juice. Add nuts. Mix and eat slowly. Chew well.

9. Fresh-Grain Breakfast (1 portion)

- 3 heaping tbsp. fresh rolled grain
- Whole milk, sour milk, or yogurt, depending on taste
- Raisins or honey, according to taste
- 1 apple, coarsely grated or 4 oz. fresh berries, or finely sliced pitted fruit
- 1 tbsp. ground hazelnuts

Moisten grain with liquids. Sweeten with raisins or honey. Add fruit and mix well. Sprinkle nuts on top.

10. Cottage Cheese-Linseed Oil Breakfast Dish (1 portion)

2 oz. cottage cheese
1 tbsp. milk or yogurt, if needed
1 tsp. linseed oil
1 tsp. lemon juice
1 tsp. honey
1 ripe banana
1 tbsp. ground linseed

If the cheese is too dry, add some of the milk or yogurt. Mix all ingredients together. Beat fruit into a froth with a fork and mix into cottage cheese and oil. Sprinkle nuts on top.

11. Small Dry Mixture (1 portion)

1 tbsp. wheat germ
1 tbsp. raisins
2 tbsp. ground hazelnuts

Mix together all ingredients. Chew thoroughly and eat slowly!

Salads, Raw Vegetables, Salad Dressings

In preparing raw vegetables, observe the following rules:

Freshness: Sun-ripened, organically grown vegetables are best, from one's own garden, if possible.

Raw vegetables should be prepared as soon as possible before eating, so that no drying or loss of juice occurs, and the chopped or sliced food comes into contact with the air as little as possible (quickly mixed with dressing or sauce).

Good quality: Leafy and tuberous vegetables should be young and tender, not pale, but full-colored, organically grown, and free of plant diseases. This is especially important for a sick person's diet.

Harmonious Combinations: Every raw-vegetable dish should consist as much as possible of the trio of tuberous, fruit, and leafy vegetables. The green leafy vegetables should never be lacking in a sick person's diet. There should also be a variety of sauces within the same raw-vegetable dish. The trio of colors enhances the beauty of the dish and contributes to the enjoyment of the meal.

Small garnishes of herbs, radishes, and new carrots, etc., can shape the raw vegetable platter festively and colorfully on special occasions. The daily trio of raw vegetables at each meal should not be exceeded; rather provide for variety in the course of the day. It is assumed that methods of cleaning vegetables are too well-known to be repeated here as well as ways of reducing their size. We recommend studying the Bircher-Benner *Eating Your Way to Health* cookbook, but other Bircher-Benner nutrition plans can often be equally helpful.

Herbs and Spices:

Fresh wild kitchen herbs are rich in vital nutrients and, in small doses, introduce a variety of taste and aroma into main dishes and raw salads. They stimulate the appetite and digestive secretions. Chopped onions, garlic, grated horseradish, ginger, cardamom, tamarind, and brewer's yeast, from a health-food store, also enrich dishes with valuable content and flavor. Sharp spices like mustard, chili, pepper, and curry should be used only in small amounts, since overstimulation of the digestive juices can cause thirst, nausea, heartburn, indigestion, and headaches.

12. Head Lettuce (Boston, iceberg)

Chives, onions, marjoram, thyme, basil

Oil dressing.

13. Leaf Lettuce (Romaine, leaf)

Chives, onions, pressed garlic if desired
Oil or yogurt dressing.

14. Endive

Chives, onions, parsley
Oil or cottage cheese-yogurt dressing.

15. Leaf Lettuce (Romaine, leaf)

Basil, marjoram
Oil or sour-milk dressing.

16. Spinach

Onions, garlic
Oil and lemon dressing.

17. Watercress

Without herbs and with onions, small amount
Oil or cottage cheese-mayonnaise dressing.

18. Spinach

Peppermint, sorrel
Oil dressing or almond-puree mayonnaise with lemon juice.

19. Cabbages

Thyme, savory, caraway seed, onions

Oil dressing; alternate also with sweet-sour sauce, with some apple concentrate or spiced cottage-cheese mayonnaise or diluted mayonnaise.

20. Savoy Cabbage

Spices and oil dressing as in recipe No. 19.

21. Red Cabbage

Wood nettle

Spices and oil dressing as in recipe No. 19.

22. Brussels Sprouts

Wood nettle

Spices and oil dressing as in recipe No. 19.

23. Chinese Cabbage

Wood nettle

Spices and oil dressing as in recipe No. 19.

24. Tomatoes

Sage, basil, thyme, dill, onion rings

Oil or yogurt dressing or diluted mayonnaise.

25. Cucumbers

Dill, borage, garlic
Oil or yogurt-cream dressing.

26. Fennel

Onions, chives
Oil or soybean-cottage cheese dressing.

27. Bell Peppers

Chives
Oil dressing.

28. Turnips

If sharp, use grated hazelnuts, no herbs
Cream or sour milk dressing.

29. Small Radishes

Chives (or without herbs)
Oil or yogurt dressing.

30. Celery Stalks

Onions, chives, parsley
Oil or soybean-cottage cheese dressing.

31. Zucchini

Dill, basil, tarragon, a little grated horseradish
Mayonnaise or spiced cottage cheese mayonnaise.

32. Carrots

Parsley, or without herbs
Garnish with hazelnuts
Yogurt or cream dressing with some honey and lemon juice.

33. Celery Root (Celeriac)

Basil, thyme, garnish with chives and walnut halves
Cream or spiced cottage cheese mayonnaise.

34. Beets

Thyme, caraway seed
Oil or cream dressing, alternate with sweet-sour sauce.

35. Cauliflower

Basil, marjoram, walnuts
Mayonnaise or spiced cottage cheese dressing.

36. Chicory

Chives, tarragon, marjoram
Sour milk or cream dressing.

37. Jerusalem Artichoke

Thyme, balm-mint
Cottage cheese-yogurt or cream dressing.

38. Kohlrabi

Thyme, or some grated horseradish
Cream or cottage cheese dressing.

39. Mixed Raw Vegetables and Appropriate Dressings

Grated, finely sliced, or chopped and mixed:
  Cucumbers, zucchini, bell peppers, tomatoes
Oil dressing.
  Cucumbers and cooked potato salad
Cream dressing.
  Chicory and apples, possibly oranges
Cottage cheese mayonnaise.
  Celery root and grated apples, nuts
Yogurt or sour-milk dressing.
  Sauerkraut and grated apples
Oil dressing.
  Chicory and diced tomatoes
Oil or mayonnaise dressing.
  Bell peppers and fennel
Oil dressing.
  Fennel and carrots, finely shredded
Oil dressing.
  Cauliflower clusters with carrots

Cream dressing.

Endive, chicory, lettuce, tomatoes

Oil dressing or mayonnaise.

Head lettuce, bell peppers, fennel, tomatoes

Oil dressing.

These mixed salads must be chewed very well. In the event of nausea, serve them without salad dressings.

40. Celery Root-Apple-Banana Raw-Food Dish
(1 portion)

1 oz. cottage cheese
3 tbsp. cream or yogurt
1/2 lemon, squeezed
7 oz. finely diced apple
4 oz. banana, sliced
2 oz. grated celery root (celeriac)
Yogurt, if needed
Walnuts

Stir together cottage cheese, cream or yogurt, lemon. Mix all ingredients together well. If too dry, add some yogurt. Garnish with walnuts.

41. Stuffed Raw Tomatoes

Horseradish
Apples
Cottage-cheese mayonnaise
Herbs
Lettuce leaves
Walnut or pineapple garnish

Grate peeled horseradish and apples into stiffly beaten cottage-cheese mayonnaise seasoned with fresh chopped herbs. Mix well, and stuff tomatoes that have been hollowed out. Place on lettuce leaves. Garnish with pieces of pineapple or walnuts on festive occasions.

42. Sauerkraut Salad

Health-food-store sauerkraut is low in salt and is a very valuable raw vegetable, especially in winter. It is more easily digestible than when cooked. When serving stewed sauerkraut, add raw sauerkraut cut into small pieces to improve the taste and digestibility.

Sauerkraut
Juniper berries
Caraway seeds
1/2 grated apple
Olive oil
Lettuce

Break up the sauerkraut, mix with some juniper berries, caraway seeds, and 1/2 grated apple, and dress with olive oil. Lettuce or any tuberous vegetable is recommended as a supplement. Sauerkraut is choleretic and stimulates the stomach and intestines.

Preparation of Raw Food:

It is important, always, first to prepare the dressing for the salads and raw vegetables, then grate, slice, or cut the carefully washed leafy or tuberous vegetables directly into the dressing and mix them together immediately. In this way, a loss in value as a result of the effect of the air on the cut vegetables can be avoided as much as possible. This is especially true of grated apples and celery root, which become discolored quickly without the dressing, but remain nice and white when mixed with the dressing. Dressed salads and raw vegetables should never be left standing for a long time, but should be eaten right away.

Salad Dressings

The following amounts are calculated for one person. Since, in general, much too much salt is used which acts as a detriment to health—especially in the case of migraine patients—all dressings for salads and fresh vegetables are to be prepared without salt. Even without salt, they can be tastily seasoned with fresh kitchen herbs, brewer's yeast extract, onions, and, if desired, crushed garlic.

43. Oil Dressing (1 portion)

1 tbsp. cold-pressed sunflower-seed oil or olive oil
1 tsp. lemon juice
1/2 tsp. finely chopped onions
1 tsp. fresh chopped herbs, or a pinch of dried herbs, or brewer's yeast extract
Garlic, possibly a very little crushed

Mix all condiments together well.

44. Cream Dressing (1 portion)

Only use this dressing if there is no sensitivity to fat.

2 tbsp. cream
1 tsp. cottage cheese
1 tsp. lemon juice
1/2 tsp. finely chopped onions, or if desired, crushed garlic
1 tsp. fresh herbs, or 1 pinch dried herbs

Beat all condiments together well with a whisk.

45. Yogurt or Sour Milk Dressing (1 portion)
(for a low-fat diet)

2-3 tbsp. yogurt, sour milk or buttermilk
A few drops lemon juice
1/2 tsp. finely chopped onions, or garlic, if desired
1 tsp. fresh herbs, or a pinch dried herbs

Mix all condiments together well.

46. Cottage-cheese-Yogurt Dressing (1 portion)

For a low-fat diet.

1 tbsp. cottage cheese
2 tbsp. yogurt or sour milk
1 tbsp. lemon juice
Fresh or dried herbs
Finely chopped onions, or crushed garlic, or
   brewer's yeast extract

Mix together thoroughly.

47. Mayonnaise (1 portion)

1 egg, beaten
1-1/4 cups oil
A few drops lemon juice
8 tbsp. vegetable bouillon, or sour milk

Add the oil drop by drop to the egg, stirring evenly with a whisk. Then dilute with vegetable bouillon or sour milk.

48. Mayonnaise Dressing (1 portion)

1 tbsp. of the mayonnaise made above
1 tsp. lemon juice
A little crushed garlic, or horseradish, if desired
1 tsp. fresh herbs, or 1 pinch dried herbs

Mix all spices well with the basic mayonnaise.

49. Soybean Mayonnaise (1 portion)

For a diet in which animal protein is forbidden.

2 level tbsp. soybean flour
3 oz. water
1 cup oil
3 tbsp. lemon juice

Stir with a whisk into a smooth paste, alternately adding water and oil to the soybean flour. Season as in Recipe No. 48.

50. Cottage-cheese Mayonnaise (1 portion)

1 tbsp. cottage cheese
1-2 tbsp. milk
1 egg yolk, if needed
1-2 tbsp. oil
1/2 tsp. dietetic mustard
1 tsp. lemon juice
Brewer's yeast extract
Fresh chopped herbs

Stir cheese and milk until smooth. Add yolk (to improve texture of sauce). Mix together all ingredients until well blended using plenty of chopped herbs.

51. Soybean-Cottage-cheese Dressing (1 portion)

1 tbsp. cottage cheese
2 tbsp. cream or yogurt
1 tsp. soybean flour
1 tsp. almond puree or tomato puree
Some onion or lemon, or salt-free spice

Mix and blend well.

52. Spiced Cottage-cheese Dressing (1 portion)

If no sensitivity to fat exists.

1 tbsp. cottage cheese
3 tbsp. yogurt, or 1 tbsp. cream and 2 tbsp. yogurt
1 tsp. soybean flour or 1 egg yolk
1 tbsp. lemon juice
Some horseradish or nutmeg and curry
1/2 apple, finely grated
Chopped watercress or chervil
1/2 tsp. fruit concentrate

Mix everything well or blend in a blender. Vary spices according to taste.

53. Sweet-Sour Dressing

For variety, every salad dressing can be made to taste sweet-sour by adding some fruit concentrate, pear juice, honey, or tomato puree. Sour milk, mixed with fruit concentrate or pear juice, also yields a low-fat dressing that is very appropriate to use with raw carrots or green lettuce.

Juices

Raw nutrition in mechanically refined form (juices), is used as supplemental special enrichment when coarse ingredients (cellulose) are forbidden such as in gastrointestinal illnesses.

Do not forget, however, that whole fresh food is always of higher value and cannot be replaced by juices over a long period of time. Therefore, return to fruit and raw vegetables as soon as possible.

In general: It is assumed that methods of cleaning and preparation are known; if not refer to *Eating Your Way to Health* by Bircher-Benner.

Many juicers are on the market for the preparation of fruit and vegetable juices, from the small hand press to the motorized centrifuge. If a hand press is used, the fruit and vegetables must first be reduced in size. Apples, pears, and all tuberous vegetables should be finely grated. Leafy vegetables and herbs should be finely chopped.

54. Fruit Juices

Serve immediately after squeezing. Letting them stand means a loss in value.

a. Unmixed fruit juices (without anything added)

Oranges, tangerines, grapefruit, apples, pears, grapes, strawberries, blueberries, currants, raspberries, peaches, apricots, plums.

b. Mixed fruit juices

Oranges, mandarin oranges, grapefruit, possibly persimmon or berry juice with apple juice or, berry juice with peach, apricot, or plum juice.

Bananas beaten together with orange, berry, peach, or apricot juice.

Depending on desire or prescription, add: lemon juice, honey, fruit concentrate, cream, yogurt, almond milk, linseed milk, rice water, or barley water (gastrointestinal illnesses).

55. Vegetable Juices

High mineral and vitamin content. Each juice has its own special value. Freshly prepared vegetable juices are basically preferred whenever possible. In addition, prepared vegetable juices of high quality are available. The best additions in this field are those obtained from lactic acid fermentation.

a. Unmixed vegetable juices:

Tomato, carrot, beet, radish, cabbage, celery, potato, all leafy, tuberous, and root vegetables.

b. Mixed vegetable juices:

From our experience, the best mixtures are carrot, tomato, spinach (in equal parts); tomato and carrot; tomato and spinach.

Other mixtures and cocktail combinations can be found, depending on individual taste.

The following may be used alternately with vegetables mentioned above: sorrel, wood nettle, chives, parsley, onions, tender celery leaves, or roots and other herbs. Add, per glass: 1/2-1 tbsp. cream, some lemon juice, perhaps some fruit concentrate, linseed milk, rice milk, and/or barley water. Other leafy vegetables or lettuces can also be used as, for example, white cabbage, cabbage, Boston lettuce, endive, Romaine lettuce, dandelion greens. In spring, the blood can be purified using stinging nettle, sorrel, and dandelion juice.

56. Potato Juice

Use well-cleaned, potatoes (peeled, if desired) (do not use unripe potatoes that have green spots, or are sprouted). Has a spasmolytic and calming effect on the stomach and intestines.

Prepare like carrot juice. The taste is not very pleasant, and this juice should be used only on a doctor's prescription: One to two tablespoons before meals, possibly mixed with another vegetable juice.

57. Puree as a Supplement to Juices

Add up to 1/3 the amount in puree to other kinds of raw juices, neutralizes sharpness of fruit taste and acids (especially beneficial for gastroenteritis and sensitivity to fruit acids).

a. Rice or barley water (puree) (1 portion)

    1 heaping tsp. rice or barley flour
    1/5 qt. water

Mix cold, boil for 5 minutes stirring constantly, let cool.

b. Linseed milk (puree) (1 portion)

Same effect as above and also easily digestible.
    1 tbsp. linseed
    1/5 qt. water

Wash and boil 10 minutes, strain and let cool. If time permits: boil for 20 minutes, doubling the amount of water—better use of linseed.

The daily amount can be prepared once daily and stored in a thermos bottle, for mixing all raw juices together.

Types of Milk

Plant Milks

58. Almond Milk and Almond Cream (for 1 portion)

This is a valuable, high-calory, vegetable protein-fat food. It reduces phlegm and has a calming effect.

    1 tbsp. almond mash
    1 tsp. honey or pear juice
    1/6 qt. water or orange juice
    For almond cream: 1/10 water

Stir almond mash and honey together with the whisk and add the water drop by drop first, until a smooth white cream is formed. Then fill glass with water or fruit juice. For almond cream, use less liquid.

59. Almond Shake (for 1 portion)

1 tbsp. almond mash
1 tsp. honey or pear juice
4 tbsp. water
8 tbsp. apple juice

Mix as above. If orange juice or apple juice is used, there is a slight thickening and more pleasant taste.

60. Sesame Milk (for 1 portion)

1 tbsp. sesame meal
1/5 qt. water
1 tsp. lemon juice
1 tsp. honey or concentrated pear juice

Mix as above.

Sesame Shake—as in Almond Shake

Cow's Milk

61. Certified Milk

Certified milk from controlled, tuberculosis-free dairies, drunk raw, is a first-rate, high quality food. It should be warmed only slightly in winter, not boiled. If unavailable, drink pasteurized, powdered, or unsweetened condensed milk.

Skim Milk: Skim milk, skimmed at home or available from the dairy or in powdered form, is highly recommended for a fat-free diet, as skim milk contains valuable milk protein, sugar, and minerals.

Whey: Whey is available fresh from the dairy or in powdered form. Whey is formed as a by-product in the preparation of cheese. It contains milk sugar, minerals (calcium, sodium, potassium) and high-quality protein ingredients (albumins). In fasts, it is an alternate to fruit juices.

Buttermilk: Buttermilk is what remains after preparing butter. It contains all milk ingredients (except fat) and is available fresh from the dairy, acidified or in powdered form. Buttermilk is easily digestible and low in calories, has a healing effect on intestinal infections, and is a very refreshing drink in summer.

62. Junket

Junket is formed from whole milk by adding rennet ferment at 98.6 degrees F. Junket is predigested whole milk, and is especially beneficial for stomach disorders and when sweet milk cannot be digested. Junket tablets are available in drug stores and health-food stores.

63. Yogurt

Yogurt is prepared by injecting warmed milk with lactic acid bacteria (acidophilia) within 6-12 hours. Yogurt is available at the dairy or can be prepared at home. It is a high-quality milk food and is easily digestible, since it is already acidified.

64. Sour Milk

Sour milk is formed by letting sweet milk stand when the weather is warm, to be acted upon by lactic acid bacteria in the air. Sour milk is especially appropriate and of great value in summer. Like yogurt, it can be enjoyed by itself or mixed with fruit.

65. Horseradish Milk (1 portion)

Mix together a small chopped apple and a small piece of horseradish, 1/2-1 inch long, depending on one's taste, fill a glass with certified milk up to about 5 ounces, and drink this beverage immediately before eating or early in the morning for stimulating the appetite. Very suitable as a refreshing drink for a sick person.

66. Kefir

Kefir is a sparkling sour milk drink, prepared from yeast mold in combination with lactic acid bacteria. They impart a pleasantly sour and tingling taste to the drink. Kefir contains valuable milk nutrients and natural carbon dioxide.

67. Milk Shakes or Yogurt Shakes (1 portion)

Nourishing, high-quality drinks can be prepared in a blender from fresh milk and fruit, in which the milk, in spite of combining with the fruit acids, does not curdle, but only thickens slightly.

About 6-8 oz. certified milk (or, if not available, pasteurized or powdered milk) mixed with 4-7 oz. fresh berries, chopped or sliced pitted fruit, or 2 oz. citrus juices, or 2 tbsp. rose hip mash.

For sweetening, instead of sugar add some honey, pear juice, or 1/2 fresh banana. In place of sweet whole milk, pleasant tasting and easily digestible shakes can be made mixed with buttermilk or sour milk or with yogurt and fruit.

If weight reduction is desired, use skimmed fresh milk or powdered milk and fill a glass with mineral water after mixing, which makes a refreshing, low-calorie drink. Without considerably increasing its nutritive value, the shake can be thickened and made to taste more pleasant by adding 2 tbsp. powdered skim milk or unsweetened condensed milk. Underweight people should drink it with some added cream, cream cheese, or an egg yolk. The nutritional value can also be increased by adding 1 tbsp. soybean milk or wheat germ. It's fun to keep trying out new combinations. Thus, for added variety, appetizing herb drinks can be created by mixing sour milk or yogurt with many minced herbs, especially dill and chives, some lemon juice, a trace of sea salt, grated cucumbers, finely diced tomatoes, or melons. These drinks are often more refreshing and digestible than sweet shakes.

68. Fortifying Drinks (1 portion)

1 tbsp. linseed
1 tbsp. almond puree
1 glass apple juice, or
1 glass orange juice
1 tsp. wheat germ
1 tsp. honey
Lemon juice, if desired
1 tbsp. rose hip mash
1 tbsp. wheat germ, or
1 tbsp. sesame meal
1 tbsp. fruit juice concentrate
6 oz. apple juice, or
another fruit juice
1 tbsp. ground almonds
Honey, if desired

Grind and soak seeds 20 minutes in water or apple juice. Add water drop by drop at first, stirring thoroughly. As soon as a white cream forms, the apple or orange juice can be poured in. Add linseed and wheat germ, sweeten to taste with some honey and give it a tang with lemon juice. Mix as in almond puree. Pour in juice and mix all spices together well. For sweetening add more honey if desired.

If sour milk is preferred, instead of apple or orange juice, sour milk, yogurt, or buttermilk can be used for variety. A small glass of such a drink to improve strength contains very high nutritive values. In case of fatigue and lack of appetite, such a drink may substitute for a meal.

Butter, Vegetable Fats, and Oils

Fresh Butter: Fresh butter is more easily digestible and improves the taste of dishes if it is added just before serving.

Vegetable Margarine and Fat: Used like butter as a spread and for improving the taste of cooked dishes, it is unsolidified, free of cholesterol, and contains unsaturated fatty acids. It is easily digestible and is used for cooking and frying. If vegetable fat is not obtainable in your health-food store, it may be prepared at home as follows:

1/3 butter
1/3 vegetable fat (nut oils)
1/3 vegetable oil

Melt butter over low heat; stir when it begins to rise until it is clear and sediment sinks. Add fat and oil. Stir until liquid and store.*

Oils: Cold-pressed oils (sunflower seed, poppy seed, olive and linseed oil, among others) are beneficial to health and should be used daily on salads and raw vegetables.

Soybean and corn oil are obtained by hot processes, but nevertheless contain valuable ingredients and are used preferably for steaming and cooking, as they are more easily digestible than heated butter and margarine.

Wheat germ oil is the richest in highly unsaturated fatty acids, but has a markedly peculiar taste. It is, therefore, mixed in spoonfuls with cottage cheese, in which its characteristic taste disappears.

Eggs and Meat

Eggs

A migraine patient should not eat any eggs at first. Later, upon recovery, he should not eat more than two a week.

Eggs must be avoided in connection with nausea. Use only fresh eggs of the very best quality; they are best used raw in drinks, softboiled, poached, or as agglutinants in creams, shakes, and mayonnaises. In this form, the vitamin and mineral content of the egg yolk is most effective. Raw egg yolk is choleretic and may therefore be eaten before eating the whole egg is permitted. Eggs are not recommended when constipated, as they promote decay. Egg protein in rather large

---

Eating Your Way to Health: The Bircher-Benner Approach to Nutrition. Baltimore, Penguin Handbooks, 1972.

amounts has an unfavorable effect on the intestinal flora. Hard-boiled eggs place stress on the liver.

Meat

Meat is not recommended for migraines, as explained on pages 22-25. It contains albumen, phosphorus, iron and other minerals. However, milk products, whole grain, and vegetables, especially soybean, nuts, potatoes, and vegetables offer a plentiful amount of high-quality protein in correct combination and, therefore, are a high-quality substitute for meat. After overcoming a migraine, cautious use of meat, if desired, is permitted, with a maximum of 2 oz. meat 2-3 times weekly.

Meat from fattened, unhealthily nourished (antibiotics and hormones) animals, pork, sausages, and shell fish should not be eaten if there is a danger of migraines.

We will not include meat recipes here, since these can be looked up in every cookbook and in connection with migraines, anyway, are used very seldom or not at all.

Cheese Recipes

Cream cheese and cottage cheese: Both cheeses are easily digestible and beneficial to intestinal flora because of their lactic-acid content. They contain abundant calcium and high-quality casein protein. As a spread for baked potatoes, and as an ideal base for fruit dishes, they are important and valuable foods that never become monotonous because of their versatility.

Soft Cheese, with fat, half-fat, and skimmed: Camembert, Bel Paese, Limburger, Gorgonzola, etc.

Soft cheeses contain salt and are harder to digest than cream cheese, but they do stimulate the appetite and are popular as an alternate spread and for baked potatoes.

Hard Cheese, fat, half-fat, skimmed: Swiss Emmentaler, Tilsit, Fontina, Parmesan, Cheddar, etc.

These cheeses have a strong taste, are spicy, stimulating to the appetite, and rich in calories, but contain salt and are harder to digest than soft and cream cheeses. If they are not forbidden by the doctor in connection with migraines and are used with restraint, they can be an alternate for whole-wheat bread, or a seasoning supplement and spread for various dishes.

69. Cottage cheese Salad Dressing (1 portion)

For a low fat diet:
    1 tbsp. cottage cheese
    2 tbsp. yogurt or sour milk
    1 tbsp. lemon juice
    Fresh or dried herbs
    Minced onions, or crushed garlic or
    Salt-free brewer's yeast

Mix all ingredients together thoroughly.

70. Cottage cheese Mayonnaise (1 portion)

    4 oz. cottage cheese
    1-2 tbsp. milk
    1 egg yolk
    1-2 tbsp. oil
    1 tsp. diet mustard
    1 tsp. lemon juice
    Some brewer's yeast
    Plenty of fresh chopped herbs

Stir cottage cheese, milk, egg, and oil until smooth. Add mustard and lemon juice to improve taste. Mix all ingredients together well.

71. Cottage cheese Fruit Creams, and Fruit Dishes (4 portions)

A fruit and cottage cheese or cream cheese dish as a dessert completes the main meal, consisting of vegetables, potatoes, or whole grain, in an ideal way because of its valuable milk protein content. Cottage cheese custards surpass other sweet dishes by their freshness, easy digestibility, and high quality. Skimmed cottage cheese can be mixed with berries, suitable fruits, or fruit juices in ever newer variations in which a few pretty berries or fruit slices serve as a garnish.

In place of sugar, it is preferable to sweeten these desserts with pear juice, honey, or a frothily beaten banana. Dates also can be used as a pleasant and healthy sweetener. For this purpose, pitted dates in vacuum-sealed packages (from the health-food store) are mashed with a fork, boiled, and strained to form date marrow.

Cream cheese Dough

Mix with preferred fresh fruit—whole, mashed, or as juice.

> 9 oz. cream or cottage cheese
> Milk or yogurt depending on taste
> 2 tbsp. pear juice, honey, or date marrow

Stir cheese and milk or yogurt until smooth. Add juice, honey or dates as sweetening.

72. Light Cottage Cheese Dumplings (Snowballs) (4 Portions)

> 14 oz. cottage cheese
> 7 oz. cream cheese
> 2 eggs
> 1 pinch sea salt
> 2 oz. flour
> 2 oz. semolina
> 3 qts. water, salted

Add all ingredients (cheese, eggs, salt, flour, semolina) one after another, to the cottage cheese, and stir well. Bring water to a boil. Dip two tablespoons into the boiling water and make large balls of the cheese dough. While placing the balls into the water, the water should not be boiling strongly, otherwise the balls will fall apart. First make a test dumpling, and, if necessary, add some semolina to the dough. Boil first uncovered for 5 min. over low heat, then 5 min. covered. Then turn each ball over once and let it sit in the water for 10 min., during which time the dumplings will still swell.

Variation:
Tomato sauce or,
stewed plums, or
stewed apricots
1 oz. melted butter
2 tbsp. toasted bread crumbs
Some raw sugar

These dumplings taste excellent in a lot of tomato sauce, or in toasted bread crumbs with some raw sugar sprinkled over them, and served with stewed plums or apricots.

73. Cottage cheese Pudding (4 portions)

1-1/2 oz. butter
4 tbsp. flour
1 pinch sea salt
1-1/4 cups hot milk
1 lb. cottage cheese
2 egg yolks
2-1/2 oz. raw sugar
1-1/2 oz. raisins
2 tbsp. ground almonds, if desired
Grated lemon peel, if desired
4 tbsp. cream, if needed
2 beaten egg whites

Sauté butter, flour, salt, together. Add milk and boil a few minutes, then let cool. Mix all ingredients together. Add cream if the mixture is too thick. Put egg whites in last. Bake in oven for 40 min. at low heat and serve immediately.

For cottage cheese cake, see Recipe 200.

74. Cottage cheese-Linseed Oil (by Dr. Budwig)
(4 portions)

11-14 oz. cream cheese
   or cottage cheese
   or a mixture of both
2 tbsp. linseed oil
2 tbsp. milk or yogurt
1 pinch seasoned salt
tomato puree or fresh tomato pulp
   or minced raw spinach or fresh herbs
Juice of 2 oranges, garnished with banana and orange circles possibly concentrated pear juice.

Mix all ingredients well. Tomato puree makes a red dish. Spinach and herbs make a green dish. Fruit makes a sweet fruit dish.

75. Cottage cheese Spread: Basic Dough
(4 portions)

For bread or as a supplement for baked potatoes. See also Bread Spreads, p. 133.

11-14 oz. cream or cottage cheese
   or a mixture of both
Some milk, if necessary

Stir until smooth.

The following seasonings are great with it:
a) Minced herbs, onions, or garlic
   Caraway seed, a pinch of seasoned salt
   Garnish with tomato slices or sliced radish

b) Plenty of chives which should be allowed to stay a while for the flavor to blend. A pinch of seasoned salt.

c) Grated raw vegetables (carrots, celery root, radish, cucumbers, etc.) seasoned depending on the different vegetables

d) Grated nuts or almonds, lemon juice, a pinch of sea salt. Garnish with chives.

Sweet Supplements:
   a) 2 tbsp. honey, 1 tsp. lemon juice
      Garnish with walnut halves
   b) 2 tbsp. fruit or pear concentrate
      Garnish: berries, fruit slices.

76. Spinach cheese or Spring Cottage Cheese Dish
(4 portions)

11-14 oz. cream or cottage cheese or a combination of both
4 tbsp. milk, if needed
2 tbsp. almond puree
4 tbsp. lemon juice
4 cups young, raw spinach, minced

Mix and stir all ingredients well. Add milk if necessary, and blend well until the mixture is smooth. If available, this dish can be supplemented by a few sorrel leaves, peppermint, watercress, chervil, or a little basil, nutmeg, or thyme. 1 pinch sea salt or seasoned salt.

Soups and Fillers

For preparing soups, sauces, and vegetables, use as much vegetable bouillon or water in its place, as possible, and a salt-free health food store vegetable-bouillion cube or vegetable paste. A good selection of fresh minced herbs gives the soup a personal touch.

If permitted, cream improves any soup and, like herbs, is added only when ready to serve. A small addition of soybean flour enriches the soup with valuable protein.

77. Vegetable Bouillon (4 portions)

2 tbsp. vegetable fat or oil
1 onion
2 carrots
5 oz. celery root
Some cabbage and Swiss chard
3-4 qts. water, cold
1 bay leaf, basil and other fresh or dried kitchen herbs. 1/2 oz. fresh butter, chives and parsley.

Can be prepared 2-3 days in advance. Cut the onion with its brown skin in half and saute the cut surface. Cut the vegetables very fine and heat at least 10 min. over a low flame, covered, steaming without water, then remove from stove. Pour on water and simmer 1-2 hrs. over a low flame. Season with herbs to taste, strain off. Add butter (if desired), chives and parsley when ready to serve.

In a normal diet, some sea salt can be added to this vegetable bouillon. Even without salt, this aromatic vegetable broth is appetizing and is usually digested well even in case of nausea.

78. Semolina as Filler (2-4 portions)

1 oz. butter
3 oz. fine semolina
1 egg
1 pinch sea salt, nutmeg

Beat butter until frothy. Mix semolina, egg, and salt well with butter and let stand for 1/2 hour, then make small balls, with two tablespoons and place them in the gently boiling bouillon for 15 min., first without cover, then allow to expand over a low flame, covered.

If a clear bouillon is desired, boil the small balls in salt water and place them in the hot bouillon when ready to serve.

79. Golden Bread Cubes as Filler (2-4 portions)

2-1/2 oz. whole-wheat bread
1 egg, beaten
3-4 tbsp. milk
1 tbsp. vegetable fat

Cut bread into equal cubes, mix egg and milk, pour over the bread and let it soak in. Bake the cubes until they are golden brown.

80. Cold Vegetable Bouillon

Cold vegetable bouillon
Ice cubes
Small cubes of peeled tomatoes, cucumbers, and bell peppers
Chopped parsley
3-1/2 oz. whipping cream (for festive occasions)

Pour bouillon into cups. Place 1 ice cube in each cup. Divide vegetables equally into cups. Top each cup with 1 tsp. whipped cream.

81. Italian Rice Soup (4 portions)

Omit cheese for a strict diet.
    1 oz. vegetable fat
    1 cup finely diced vegetables (carrots, onions, celery root)
    14 oz. spinach, finely chopped
    5 oz. rice
    2 qt. lightly salted vegetable broth
    2-3 tbsp. grated Parmesan cheese

Melt fat. Sauté vegetables until they have changed color. Add spinach. Add rice, broth, and cook for 20 min. Sprinkle cheese over soup in bowls, if desired.

82. Soybean Soup (4 portions)

2 tbsp. vegetable fat
1/2 onion, chopped
4-5 tbsp. flour
1 tbsp. soybean flour
1 peeled tomato, diced
2 qts. vegetable bouillon
1 pinch sea salt
2 tbsp. cream
Chives, parsley

Sauté onion in fat lightly. Add flour stirring until smooth. Add tomato and pour bouillon over all. Boil 1/2 hour and strain. Add salt, chives, parsley and, last, cream.

83. Potato Soup (4 portions)

1 tbsp. vegetable fat
1/2 chopped onion
1 leek
7 oz. celery
1 small carrot
4 medium-sized potatoes
1 tbsp. whole meal
1 tsp. soybean flour
2 qts. water or vegetable broth
1 pinch sea salt
2 tbsp. cream or milk
Chopped marjoram
Chives

Melt fat and saute onion briefly. Cut up vegetables very fine and add. Sprinkle flour over the mixture and saute all together for a few minutes. Pour broth over all, boil 1/2 hr. and strain. Add salt, marjoram, chives and cream and serve.

The following soups should be made only in nonfat vegetable bouillon and 1 tsp. vegetable fat or oil added just prior to serving (if a strict nonfat diet is not required).

84. Sago Soup with Vegetable Filler
(4 portions)

2 oz. sago
2 qts. boiling vegetable broth
2 tsp. vegetable fat
4 small carrots
2 pieces celery root, average size
1 leek
1 pinch salt

Stir sago into the boiling vegetable broth; cut carrots and celery root into small cubes, and leek into fine strips. Sauté well in vegetable fat; add to vegetable broth and cook 1/2 hour (or omit vegetables and season with chives).

85. Clear Rice Soup (4 portions)

1 chopped onion
4 tbsp. finely chopped vegetables (carrots, celery root, leek)
4 tbsp. rice
2 qts. vegetable broth (hot)
1 tsp. vegetable fat
Chives

Steam vegetables and rice in small amount of broth. Add rest of hot vegetable broth and cook for at least 20 min. Place fat and chives in bowls and add hot soup to serve.

86. Rice Cream Soup (4 portions)

2 qts. vegetable broth (more if needed)
3 oz. rice flour
2 tsp. whole wheat flour
Cold water (small amount)
1 pinch salt
2 level tsp. vegetable fat (health store)
4 tbsp. cream
Chives, to taste

Bring stock to a boil. Combine flours and salt with just enough cold water to make a smooth creamy consistency. Add to the boiling broth with salt. Cook 1/2 hr. stirring to prevent sticking. Place fat, cream, chives in bowls, and pour soup over all, to serve.

87. Cream Soup (4 portions)

8 level tbsp. whole wheat flour
2 qts. vegetable broth
3/4 cup milk
1 pinch salt
2 tsp. vegetable fat
4 tbsp. cream
Chives, nutmeg

Prepare as in recipe 86.

88. Herb Soup

Prepare as cream soup and add fresh or dried herbs, such as basil, tarragon, etc., to taste.

89. Cream of Oat Soup (4 portions)

1/2 cup rolled oats
2 qts. vegetable broth
2 pieces celery root
1 pinch salt
2 tsp. vegetable fat
4 tbsp cream, if desired
Chives, if desired

Prepare as in recipe 86.

90. Oat Porridge Soup (4 portions)

8 tbsp. rolled oats
2 qts. cold water
Salt, to taste
1 tsp. vegetable fat

Boil 30-40 min, in water (possibly with some salt) and strain. Add fat to soup to improve taste.

91. Oatmeal Soup (4 portions)

1 tsp. health food store vegetable fat
8 tbsp. oatmeal
1-1/2-2 qts. vegetable broth
3/4 cup milk
1 pinch salt
Chives

Sauté oatmeal in vegetable fat, add vegetable broth, milk and salt, and cook 30 minutes. Add chives before serving.

92. Oat Groats Soup (4 portions)

2 tsp. vegetable fat
8 tbsp. groats
2 qts. water
1-1/4 cups milk
2 small slices celery root
1 pinch salt
Yeast extract

Sauté oat grits lightly in vegetable fat. Add water, milk, celery and salt and cook 1 hr. Add yeast extract to soup just before serving.

93. Barley Soup (4 portions)

2 tsp. health food store vegetable fat.
1/2 chopped onion
1 minced leek
4 small carrots
4 slices celery root, minced
4 oz. barley
12 tbsp. water
3/4-1-1/2 cups milk
1 pinch salt
Nutmeg, chives, to taste

Melt fat and sauté onion, leeks, carrots, celery root lightly. Add barley, water, milk, and salt, and cook 1 hr., stirring occasionally. Add nutmeg and chives to soup before serving.

94. Nonfat Tomato Soup (4 portions)

16 ripe tomatoes
1 pinch salt
1 qt. vegetable broth
1 tsp. sugar (if desired)
Herbs and lemon juice, to taste

Cut tomatoes into pieces, add salt and cook briefly in vegetable broth. Add remaining ingredients and heat briefly.

95. Tomato Soup (4 portions)

2 tsp. vegetable fat
4 small carrots
4 small pieces celery root
1 leek
Some rosemary
8 tomatoes
2 tbsp. flour
1-1/2 qt. vegetable broth
1 pinch salt
Chives

Melt fat. Cut up carrots, celery root, leek and sauté well in the vegetable fat. Add tomatoes and mix. Sprinkle flour over vegetables and add the broth slowly. Cook 10 min. Add chives to soup before serving.

96. Raw Tomato Soup (4 portions)

4-6 ripe juicy tomatoes per person
Apple juice, to taste
1 tbsp. lemon juice per person
Finely minced rosemary
1 pinch sea salt
Basil or nutmeg
2 tbsp. yogurt or cream per person
Crispbread, with butter or cream cheese spread, if desired.

Cut up tomatoes and strain. Add apple juice to taste and stir. Mix remaining ingredients together and add to tomato mixture. Crispbread may be used as an accompaniment to the soup.

97. Carrot Soup (4 portions)

2 tsp. vegetable fat
1/2 chopped onion
4 cut carrots
2 tbsp. flour
1-1/2 qts. vegetable broth
2 cups milk (about)
1 pinch salt
1/4 tsp. caraway seeds
Celery leaves

Melt fat. Sauté onion and carrots in vegetable fat. Sprinkle flour over vegetables, sauté lightly. Add broth, milk, and salt, cook 1/2 hr. Strain. Add caraway seeds and celery leaves to soup before serving.

98. Spinach or Swiss Chard Soup (4 portions)

2 tsp. vegetable fat
4 tbsp. flour
2 plates chopped spinach
1-1/2 qts. vegetable broth
2 tsp. spinach leaves
Nutmeg, 8 leaves peppermint

Sauté flour in vegetable fat. Add spinach and sauté in flour and fat. Add broth to spinach mixture, and cook 20 min. Blend or mince spinach and peppermint and add to the finished soup. (Do not continue to cook.)

99. Celery Soup (4 portions)

4 tsp. vegetable fat
4 small celery roots, minced
4 tbsp. flour
2 qts. vegetable broth
1 pinch salt
Bay leaf, nutmeg

Sauté celery in melted vegetable fat. Sprinkle flour over celery and sauté. Add broth, salt, herbs and cook 3/4 hr. Strain before serving.

100. Chervil Soup (4 portions)

4 potatoes, diced
4 tsp. flour
Salt
2 qts. vegetable broth
3-4 level tsp. chopped chervil

Stew potatoes in vegetable broth and salt, cook 1/2 hr. and strain. Add chervil to the soup before serving.

101. Spring Soup (4 portions)

4 tbsp. flour
2 qts. water or vegetable broth
Salt
1 onion
4 young carrots
Small celery leaves
A few spinach leaves
Sorrel, wood nettle leaves or dandelion leaves
3/4 cup milk

Stir flour into vegetable broth. Cook 1/2 hr. Chop vegetables fine, add, and let stand a few minutes. Add milk to soup.

102. Potato Soup (4 portions)

2 leeks, cut up
4 slices celery root
2 young carrots
4 large potatoes, cut into pieces
4 level tbsp. flour
2 qt. vegetable broth
1 pinch salt
Marjoram and chives

Stew leeks, celery root, carrots, potatoes, in a little vegetable broth. Sprinkle flour over vegetables. Add rest of broth and salt, and cook 1/2 hr. Strain. Add herbs to soup before serving.

103. Cheese Soup (if cheese is permitted) (4 portions)

1-2 tbsp. vegetable fat
5 tbsp. whole wheat flour
1 tbsp. white flour
3 tbsp. soybean flour
1-1/2 qts. water or vegetable broth
1 whole onion, with 1 bay leaf held in place by 2 cloves
2 oz. Parmesan cheese
1 cup milk
Chives, parsley, possibly some tarragon
Salt

Melt fat. Sauté flour lightly in fat. Add water or broth, stir. Add onion, and cook 20-30 min. over a low flame. Stir grated cheese and milk together and add herbs with salt if desired. Pour hot soup over everything.

Cooked Vegetables

Steamed vegetables are very nutritious because they contain carbohydrates, vegetable protein, minerals, aromatic substances, and vitamins. In steaming, they retain their nutritional values, nourish without burdening the digestion, are low in calories but rich in cellulose, and are, therefore, satisfying without being fattening, and also stimulate the intestines.

It is important to buy fresh, organically grown vegetables. When unavailable, frozen vegetables, without preservatives, can be used.

Cabbage, spinach, viper's grass, and legumes can cause flatulence, but are very rich in valuable nutrients.

If diarrhea exists, legumes that cause flatulence must be avoided. Sauerkraut and spinach have a laxative effect. Carrots, tomatoes, lettuce, beets, celery, artichokes, chicory, and fennel are most easy to digest.

The same basic rules apply for preparing vegetables as for raw food: freshness, quality, cleanliness, and care.

Almost all vegetables can be gently steamed or stewed in their own juices or with a little water in a heavy pan and tightly covered over a low flame. All nutrients are best retained in this kind of preparation. The food is also tastier than vegetables that are cooked in salt water and lose their nutritive power. When vegetables must be cooked briefly in salt water (as for example, cauliflower) or, better, cooked gently in a collander over boiling water, the cooking water can be used for sauces or soups. Asparagus is an exception, since the water that asparagus is cooked in is not beneficial to health.

Cooking time, quantity, and weight cannot always be given exactly in the following recipes, as the vegetables vary in freshness, size, and quality. If a pressure cooker is used, look up the cooking times.

Some ingredients can be omitted or replaced by others, depending entirely on taste. It is important, however, to use very little salt. By carefully measuring the amount of herbs, salt is easily replaceable. After a short period of adjustment to the new diet, you will find that the delicate individual taste of lightly salted vegetables is most enjoyable.

104. Spinach, Whole Leaves (4 portions)

Especially valuable for its iron and chlorophyll content.

2 lbs. spinach (when possible, use young, tender leaves)
2 tbsp. vegetable fat
1 small chopped onion
1 chopped garlic clove
1 pinch sea salt
Nutmeg
1/2 oz. butter

Remove stems and wash thoroughly. Coarse winter spinach must be placed briefly in boiling salt water; if the water tastes bitter, do not use it again. Melt fat. Sauté onion and garlic gently. Add spinach and steam for a short time over a low flame, until done. Add salt and nutmeg before serving, topped with butter.

105. Chopped Spinach (4 portions)

2 lbs. spinach
1 tbsp. vegetable fat
1 small chopped onion
1 chopped garlic clove
1 tsp. whole wheat flour
1 tsp. white flour
3/4 cup milk or spinach broth (if not bitter)
1 pinch sea salt
Nutmeg
4 oz. raw spinach
A few peppermint leaves or sorrel leaves
2 tbsp. cream.

Remove thick stems, wash thoroughly. Steam, covered, over a low flame, until the spinach has absorbed water. Then chop fine or put through chopping machine. Keep broth. Melt fat. Sauté together onion and garlic. Sprinkle flour over onion. Pour milk over flour and onion and cook 15 min. Then add the chopped spinach and cook a little longer. Mince or blend raw spinach and add before serving. Do not cook. Add cream to the mixture.

106. Spinach Pudding (4 portions)

1-1/2 oz. butter or vegetable fat
1 chopped onion
1 tbsp. chopped herbs
1-1/2 oz. whole wheat flour
1/2 oz. white flour
12 tbsp. cold milk
1/2 tsp. sea salt
9 oz. spinach
3-4 egg yolks
Nutmeg
3-4 egg whites, stiffly beaten
Caper sauce

Sauté together butter or fat and onion. Add herbs and saute. Mix in flour. Pour milk over mixture and cook until it is thick. Add salt. Wash, mince, and add spinach to the cooled sauce. Stir in yolks and nutmeg, and mix together well. Carefully fold in egg whites. Grease and flour a pudding mold. Fill spinach into pudding mold and cook in a double-boiler for 1 hour. Unmold on a hot plate. Serve sauce with pudding.

107. Lettuce (4 portions)

4 medium-sized heads of lettuce
2 tbsp. vegetable fat
1 small chopped onion
1 pinch sea salt
1/4 qt. vegetable broth
3 tbsp. cream or milk

Cut lettuce heads in half; cook gently until medium soft. Drain, and remove to a heat-resistant dish, filling it. Melt fat. Sauté onion golden brown in vegetable fat and spread over the lettuce. Add salt and broth, and bake 30 min. in oven. Pour cream over lettuce before serving.

108. Endive (4 portions)

2-4 endive heads
2 tbsp. vegetable fat
1 small chopped onion
1 pinch sea salt
2 tbsp. cream or milk

Prepare endive like lettuce, wash, cut into fine strips. Sauté onion in vegetable fat, add endive strips, and sauté gently, covered, over a low flame. Pour cream or milk over endives before serving.

109. Chicory (slightly bitter, choleretic) (4 portions)

1-3/4 lbs. prepared chicory
1 tbsp. vegetable fat or oil
4 tbsp. milk or cream
8 tbsp. vegetable broth
1 pinch sea salt
A few drops of lemon juice, if desired
Butter, melted, if desired

Cut chicory into wedges. Melt fat. Place the chicory in layers in the saucepan. Add milk, broth, and salt, cover and stew gently for 1 hr. over a low flame. Pour lemon juice and hot melted butter over the chicory when ready to serve.

110. Vegetable Jelly (by Dr. Dorschner) (4 portions)

Sauteed, chopped mixed vegetables (carrots, celery, cauliflower, beans, etc.)
1 qt. vegetable broth
1 tbsp. agar-agar powder
Seasoned salt, chopped garlic
A few drops lemon juice

Fill a cup or small mold with vegetables. Heat broth and agar-agar to 140-176 degrees with seasoning, as listed. Pour the hot liquid over the vegetables and let cool. Pour the whole mass out on plate, garnish with parsley, serve.

111. Baked Tomatoes and Eggplant (4 portions)

2 tbsp. oil
1/2 onion, chopped
1-1/2 lb. eggplant
1 pinch sea salt
7 oz. tomatoes
Thyme, basil
1 sage leaf
1 tbsp. flour
1 tsp. Parmesan cheese
1 tsp. Gruyere cheese

Melt oil. Saute onion in oil. Cut eggplant, unpeeled, into strips 1/2 in. thick. Sauté with onion, very briefly, to prevent the strips from falling apart. Dip tomatoes into boiling water, peel, cut into large slices, then sauté with eggplant. Cook spices with vegetables. Sprinkle flour over mixture. Grate cheese and sprinkle over vegetables. Place together in a heat-resistant dish and bake for a short time in broiler until a small brown crust has formed.

112. Stuffed and Baked Tomatoes (4 portions)

8 small or 4 large tomatoes
8 tsp. cooked whole long-grain rice
1 pinch salt
Chopped basil
1 chopped garlic clove
2 tbsp. oil for heat-resistant dish

Cut off tops, reserving them; hollow out tomatoes, strain the pulp and mix with rice and spices. Fill the tomatoes, place pats of butter on top, and replace tomato tops. Arrange in heat-resistant dish and bake at medium temperature for 20-30 min.

113. Rice Filling for Stuffed Tomatoes or Stuffed Eggplant

3 tbsp. whole long-grain rice
1 cup vegetable broth
1 pinch sea salt
1 egg
2 tbsp. grated cheese
Fresh chopped herbs
2 tbsp. chopped mushrooms

Boil broth and rice gently until rice is cooked. Mix all ingredients with the rice and fill hollowed out tomatoes or eggplant. Bake in oven until eggplant or tomatoes are soft.

114. Zucchini (4 portions)

1-3/4 lb zucchini squash
2 tbsp. vegetable fat or oil
1 small chopped onion
1 pinch sea salt
Rosemary, dill, parsley, basil
7 oz. tomatoes
1 tsp. corn starch, dissolved in a little cold water

Dice zucchini unpeeled, or cut into thick strips. Melt fat. Sauté onion, salt, and spices together. Dip tomatoes into boiling water, peel, cut up, add to the half-softened zucchini and bake together until ready. If too much liquid has formed, add cornstarch paste to mixture.

115. Eggplant (4 portions)

About 1-3/4 lbs. eggplant
2 tbsp. vegetable fat
1 pinch salt
Vegetable broth, if needed

Wash, peel, and cut eggplant into cubes. Sauté until soft. Garnish with some steamed tomato halves or plum tomatoes.

116. Artichokes (slightly choleretic) (4 portions)

Cut the stalks off the artichokes, remove the lower hard leaves, and cut off the tips. Cut in half, cut off blooms, wash under running water.

2 large (or 4 small) artichokes
2 qt. salt water
1 tsp. lemon juice

Bring to a boil and boil gently for about 3/4 hr. Drain and serve on a warm dish covered with a napkin. Serve with Hollandaise, Remoulade, or Vinaigrette sauce. Cottage cheese sauce is easy on the liver (cottage cheese mixed with yogurt) and herbs and brewer's yeast improve the taste.

116. Bell Peppers Stuffed with Rice (4 portions)

4 large peppers
2 qts. salt water
1 tbsp. vegetable fat
1/2 chopped onion
1/2 chopped garlic clove
4-1/2 oz. rice
5 oz. tomatoes
1 pinch sea salt
12-16 tbsp. vegetable broth
1-1/2 tbsp. butter
1/2 oz. grated cheese
1/2 qt. tomato sauce

Cut off stems, take out seeds, and boil peppers in salt water until medium soft. Melt fat. Sauté onion and garlic together. Add the rice and sauté. Peel tomatoes, dice, add with salt, and cook 18 min. Add broth to rice last. Stuff the prepared tomato rice into the precooked peppers (not too full, so the peppers do not split). Place the stuffed peppers in a heat-resistant casserole dish, fill with tomato sauce, and sprinkle with cheese. Dot top with butter. Bake about 1/2 hr., possibly pour some more sauce over.

117. Pepperonata (4 portions)

4 tbsp. oil
1 small chopped onion
7 oz. bell peppers
7 oz. zucchini
1 pinch sea salt
7 oz. eggplant
7 oz. tomatoes
1 tbsp. whole wheat flour
1 tsp. grated Parmesan cheese
1 tsp. grated Gruyere cheese

Heat oil. Sauté onion. Cut peppers in half, remove seeds, cut into rectangles. Cut unpeeled zucchini into 1/2-1 inch slices; sauté with peppers until medium soft. Cut eggplant like zucchini. Dip tomatoes into boiling water and peel, then cut into large pieces and mix with eggplant and other vegetables. Sprinkle flour over vegetables to thicken the vegetable juices, which will be plentiful. Sprinkle cheese over the vegetables when ready to serve.

118. Chicory (4 portions)

2 lbs. prepared chicory
8 tbsp. milk
1/5 qt. vegetable broth
1 pinch salt
A few drops lemon juice, if desired

Place in saucepan (stem cut into cross sections). Add milk and broth, and cook, covered, over low heat for 15 min. Season to taste with salt and a little lemon juice.

119. Celery (4 portions)

2 lbs. celery
2 cups vegetable broth
A few drops lemon juice
Or, 2 tbsp. milk
1 pinch salt

Cut celery into about 3-inch long pieces. Add lemon juice and milk and cook gently, covered, for 1/2-1 hr. over a low flame.

120. Cooked Carrots (4 portions)

2 lbs. carrots (cut in slices or shredded)
2 cups vegetable broth
1 pinch salt
Rosemary

Cook carrots for 20-30 min. in broth with salt and rosemary.

121. Fennel (4 portions)

2-3 rather large stalks of fennel
8 tbsp. milk
1/5 qt. vegetable broth
1 pinch salt

Cut in half and wash (cut away tough parts). Add milk and broth with salt, and stew gently, covered, for 3/4 hr.

122. Sweet Peas and Carrots (4 portions)

1 lb. shelled peas
1 lb. carrots (prepared)
1 cup vegetable broth
A little onion
1 pinch salt

Prepare peas as in following recipe. Cut carrots into fine strips and prepare as in the cooked-carrots recipe (120). Add salt and mix peas and carrots in the saucepan; or, serve separately.

123. Peas (4 portions)

2 lbs. only very young, shelled sweet peas
2/5 qt. vegetable broth
1 pinch salt

Cook peas in broth over a very low flame until peas are soft, 20-30 min., depending on quality. Add salt.

124. Steamed Celery Root (Celeriac) (4 portions)

2 lbs. celery root
A few drops lemon juice
Or, 2 tbsp. milk
2 cups vegetable broth
1 pinch salt

Cut celery root in small rectangles and cook 1/2-3/4 hr. in milk, broth and salt.

125. Red Beets (4 portions)

1-1/2 lbs. beets
Salt water
2 tsp. vegetable fat
2 grated apples
1 cup vegetable broth
1 small pinch sugar
A few drops lemon juice
1 small bay leaf
1 pinch caraway seed
1 pinch salt

Cut off root tips and leaves of beets leaving about 3/4 inch, wash well, without damaging the surface. Cook gently in salt water for 2-3 hrs. (about 25 min. in pressure cooker). Pour cold water over all, peel beets, and cut into fine slices. Bring to boil vegetable broth and beet juice in equal parts. Add grated apple, thicken with some corn starch, if desired, and add seasoning. Cook Briefly.

126. Jerusalem Artichokes (4 portions)

3/4 lb. Jerusalem artichokes
Water
1 pinch salt
Vegetable broth
Basil

Brush and wash artichokes, and place in a sieve or collander. Set in pan and add water and salt up to holes of container. Cover pan and cook 30-40 min. Peel artichokes and cut in slices. Stew in vegetable broth and seasonings.

127. Mixed Vegetables (4 portions)

1 tbsp. vegetable fat
1 onion, chopped
1-2 pieces zucchini (about 1/2 lb.)
1-2 pieces eggplant (about 1/2 lb.)
1-2 tomatoes
1 pinch salt
1-2 potatoes

Melt fat, and sauté onion. Cut zucchini and eggplant in half, remove seeds, and cut into cubes. Peel and cut tomatoes into large cubes. Add salt for seasoning. Cut potatoes into 1/2-inch cubes; add and cook all together 1/2 hr. If too much juice forms, simmer uncovered, until it is desired consistency.

128. Broccoli (4 portions)

If permitted and digestible:
   1 broccoli branch
   1/2 qt. salt water
   Vegetable fat
   Or, tomato sauce

Cut off leaves and trunk under crowns, cut into rather large pieces, peel trunk parts, retain tender leaves, soak 1 hr. in cold salt water, then rinse well. Boil broccoli in water 20-30 min. Serve in a hot deep dish. Heat, but do not brown, fat and pour over broccoli.

Potato Dishes

129. Boiled Unpeeled Potatoes (4 portions)

White and red potatoes are best.
   8 average-sized potatoes
   Salt water

Brush and wash potatoes. Put potatoes into collander and set in pan. Add water up to holes of colander, cover, and cook gently 30-40 min.

130. Baked Potatoes (4 portions)

   8 average-sized potatoes
   1-1/2 tsp. oil
   1 pinch salt

Brush and wash. Cut 3-4 slits in top side of potatoes. Brush potatoes, with oil. Season and bake at average heat 30-40 minutes on a greased cookie sheet. Place a small pat of fat on each of the prepared potatoes (if permitted).

131. Potatoes with Cottage Cheese (4 portions)

8 average-sized potatoes
1 pinch salt
1-1/2 tsp. oil
Filling:
    7 oz. cottage cheese
    4-6 tbsp. milk or cream
    Chives or caraway seeds or marjoram

Cut a ridge in the top side of the potatoes and prepare as in baked potatoes. Stir cottage cheese and milk until frothy and mix with the other ingredients. Dress potatoes by forcing filling through pastry tube over the ridge of the baked potatoes.

132. Caraway Seed Potatoes (4 portions)

6-8 average-sized potatoes (rather long, thin)
Some caraway seed
1 pinch salt
Some oil

Brush potatoes, wash, and cut in half down the middle. Mix and sprinkle salt and caraway seeds on the cut surface of the potatoes. Place the cut surface down on a lightly greased cookie sheet and bake at average heat for 3/4 hr.

133. Bouillon Potatoes (4 portions)

8 potatoes
3 cups lightly salted vegetable broth
Vegetable fat, small amount

Wash potatoes, peel, and cut in halves or in pieces and cook gently. Let fat melt over small pieces of potato when ready to serve (if permitted).

134. Parsley Potatoes (4 portions)

8 peeled potatoes
1 pinch salt
A little water
Some vegetable fat
4 tsp. chopped parsley

Prepare potatoes—wash and peel. Divide them into 4 pieces lengthwise. Sprinkle them with salt. Cook potatoes in colander or sieve over steam. Let fat melt, mix parsley and potatoes with it and serve.

135. Milk Potatoes (4 portions)

About 1-1/2 lbs. potatoes
3/4 cup vegetable broth
4 tbsp. buttermilk or skim milk
1 pinch salt
Parsley

Cut potatoes in slices, steam for a short time and cook gently in vegetable broth and milk with salt. Sprinkle parsley over potatoes.

136. Potatoes with Tomatoes (4 portions)

1-1/2 lbs. potatoes
3/4 cup vegetable broth
1 pinch salt
About 1 lb. tomatoes

Peel potatoes, cut into slices, and cook until medium soft in vegetable broth with salt. Peel tomatoes, cut into small cubes, add and cook until done.

137. Potato Goulash (4 portions)

4-5 average sized onions, minced
Oil
6-8 average sized potatoes
Chopped parsley

Sauté onions in oil. Cut potatoes into slices, add enough water so it won't burn and cook thoroughly, covered. Add salt, marjoram, and parsley for seasoning.

138. Potato Snow (4 portions)

8 average-sized potatoes
1 pinch salt
Water
Vegetable fat

Peel and cut potatoes into pieces, cook (steam) with a little water until soft. Press through a potato press directly onto a warm plate. Place fat in small pats over potatoes.

139. Mashed Potatoes (4 portions)

8 average-sized potatoes
A little water
1 pinch salt
2 oz. health food store vegetable fat
2/5 qt. milk or buttermilk or
Skimmed milk
Some nutmeg
Parsley

Peel potatoes, cut into pieces, steam in a little water until soft, strain through a potato press, colander, sieve or masher. Warm vegetable fat and milk, add to potatoes, and beat until frothy. Add nutmeg for seasoning. Serve on a hot plate. Dip knife in hot water and make patterns on potatoes. Garnish with parsley.

140. Potato Cakes (4 portions)

About 2 lbs. raw potatoes, grated
Water
1 egg
Some soybean flour
1 minced onion
Some seasoned salt, caraway seed, garlic, fine marjoram, tarragon, dandelion, plantain, watercress
About 1 tbsp. whole grain flour
A little oil

Peel and grate potatoes. Prepare a dough by mixing egg, soybean flour, onion, salt and herbs. Add flour and oil, depending on the consistency of the dough. Form flat cakes about the size of the palm of the hand, and bake on both sides.

141. Potatoes in Aluminum Foil (4 portions)

1-3/4 lbs. potatoes
1 tsp. oil
Aluminum foil for wrapping
Some butter or cream cheese or sour cream
Chopped chives

Brush and wash potatoes under hot running water. Dry. Brush potatoes with oil. Wrap each potato in aluminum foil. Bake in oven at high heat for 30-40 min. Open the foil only when ready to mash the potatoes and cream cheese or sour cream with 2 forks in their crisp jackets. Sprinkle chives on top.

Grain and Meal*

142. Uncooked (4 portions)

7 oz. ground wheat, oats, rye, barley, or millet
Water or apple juice
1 pinch sea salt or
4 tsp. fruit concentrate or,
4 tsp. honey or,
Grated lemon peel
About 1/2 cup (or more) milk per person

Use grain that has been organically grown, if possible, and grind at home with a special mill, or have it done at a health-food store. Soak for 6-12 hours. The liquid should only just cover the grain and should be absorbed during the soaking. Add salt, fruit concentrate or honey, and lemon peel as seasoning. Pour milk over gain to taste.

143. Cooked and Seasoned

7 oz. coarsely ground wheat grains
1 qt. water or vegetable broth
Vegetable fat or,
    2-4 tbsp. grated cheese or
    stewed onion rings, if desired
Kitchen herbs to taste

Soak grain 6-12 hrs. Then cook for about 10 min. over very low heat or preferably in a double boiler. Do not add salt. Pour or sprinkle fat over the prepared gruel. Add cheese and herbs.

---

*Observe special instructions when cooking in a pressure cooker.

144. Sweet Whole-wheat, cooked in milk (4 portions)

7 oz. ground wheat
2 cups water
2 cups milk
2 tbsp. semolina (farina) or ground millet
1/2 oz. butter or vegetable fat
Compote of apples or prunes or honey or raisins.

Do not soak the wheat, to keep it from becoming pasty; pour boiling water (possibly 1 pinch salt) over the wheat, and cook until semi-soft and water is absorbed, let it swell for 30 min. while covered, then pour boiling milk over the grain and finish cooking. Total cooking time, about 1 hr. Top with butter and serve with compote.

145. Whole Wheat dish (like Rissotto) (4 portions)

1 cup ground whole wheat (about 7 oz.)
1 tbsp. vegetable fat
1 chopped onion
3 cups vegetable broth
1 pinch sea salt
Pats of butter
2 tbsp. grated cheese or plenty of chives

Melt fat. Sauté wheat and onion in fat. Bring broth to a boil and pour boiling over wheat. Let wheat swell, at low heat or, preferably, in the oven for 20 min. Place pats of butter on the wheat. Add cheese and/or chives. Like Risotto, ground wheat can also be prepared with diced vegetables, peas, and mushrooms and also enriched with steamed tomatoes.

146. Ground Wheat Pudding (4 portions)

9 oz. ground wheat
About 1 qt. water
1 pinch sea salt
1 small leek
3 egg yolks
Grated lemon peel, if desired
3 egg whites
4 oz. grated cheese or onion rings sauteed golden brown in butter according to taste
Supplement with juicy steamed vegetables, steamed tomatoes, or tomato or herb sauce

Presoak wheat for 6 hrs. and cook for 10 min. with salt; or cook 30-40 min. with salt without presoaking. Chop leek fine, cook with wheat. Let the prepared gruel cool. Beat egg yolks and fold in. Beat egg whites until stiff, and fold in carefully. Fill buttered mold with the mixture in layers alternating with grated cheese. (The cheese can also be omitted and a layer of sautéed onion rings can be inserted between the layers of ground grain instead.) Bake in a preheated oven about 30 min., until a light-brown crust has formed.

147. Corn Flakes with Fruit and Milk
(If no intolerance to milk exists)

Different grain flakes with fresh whole milk makes a popular summer dish. Yogurt, sour, and buttermilk are better suited to mixing with berries and fruit, since they do not curdle as whole milk does, in the process. Dried figs, plums, or pears cut into small pieces, presoaked in apple juice, and placed in layers in sour milk or yogurt make a nourishing, refreshing dish that promotes digestion.

148. Sprouted Cereal Grains

Especially high content in vitamin E and B complex, this method of eating grains has a fortifying effect. To sprout them follow these directions:

1st day, evening: Wash the seeds of grain in a colander under the tap or running water and place in a small bowl. Cover with water. Let stand at room temperature or near the oven.

2nd day, morning: Rinse seed grains and spread out on a flat plate, to dry at room temperature or near the oven. Evening: Place in a small bowl and cover again with water. Let stand at room temperature, or near oven.

3rd day, morning: Rinse off seeds and spread out to dry on a plate. Evening: Place in a small bowl and cover with water, at room temperature, or near oven. The seeds should have developed sprouts about 1 inch long.

149. Buckwheat Groats (4 portions)

Buckwheat is a very valuable cereal that contains rutin. Rutin strengthens capillary blood vessels as in hypertension and in radiation injury.

1 cup buckwheat (about 7 oz.)
1 tbsp. oil
2 cups water
1 pinch sea salt
1/2 oz. butter
1/2 qt. sour milk or beaten yogurt

Wash and sauté with oil in a frying pan until the buckwheat is slightly brown. Boil water and add, with salt, to the sautéed buckwheat. Simmer for 20 min. covered over a low flame. Place pat of butter on each dish of prepared buckwheat. Add yogurt or milk to dish.

150. Baked Buckwheat Groats (4 portions)

2 cups buckwheat
4 cups water
1 pinch salt
1/2 oz. vegetable fat (to grease pudding mold and for flakes)

Soak buckwheat for 24 hrs. Steam with salt (in a well-covered pan) for 1 hr. or bake in oven in a greased pudding mold covered, set in boiling water, for 1 hr., until upper surface is dry. Also serve with cold milk or yogurt or buttermilk. Add some honey and vegetable fat if desired.

151. Mock Meat Loaf made of Ground Spelt (green rye)

9 oz. ground green spelt
2/5 qt. cold water
1 tbsp. oil
1-1/2 oz. chopped onion
4 oz. chopped mushrooms
1 tbsp. chopped parsley
Marjoram, brewer's yeast, 1 pinch sea salt
1/2 oz. grated Parmesan cheese
2 eggs
1 tbsp. rolled oats, if needed

Let spelt swell in water over a low flame for 45 min. Sauté the onions in oil first, then add and sauté the mushrooms and parsley and mix with the spelt. If the mixture is too soft, add some rolled oats.

Mix all ingredients together, and form a meat loaf. Place in a heat-resistant dish.

Sauce:
1 tbsp. oil
1 large chopped onion
1 lb. tomatoes
1/2 oz. butter patties

First cook the onions and then the tomatoes, strain, and pour over the meat loaf. Place butter patties on the dish. Bake 1/2 hr. in a preheated oven at medium heat while basting several times with tomato sauce.

152. Spelt Mash (by Dr. Dorschner) (4 portions)

    1 cup green spelt (about 7 oz.)
    2 cups water
    1 minced onion
    Seasoned or celery salt, chopped garlic, marjoram, cold-pressed sunflower seed oil and plenty of minced herbs

Grind spelt in a blender or coffee mill. Cook about 20 minutes with onion in water (a pressure cooker is best). Season with salt, herbs and sunflower-seed oil.

153. Millet Risotto (4 portions)

    1 tbsp. vegetable fat
    1 small chopped onion
    7 oz. millet
      (corn, semolina, buckwheat, spelt)
    2/3 qt. boiling vegetable broth
    1 pinch sea salt
    2 tbsp. grated cheese or
    1/2 oz. butter and
    1/2 onion, cut into strips
    Supplement: tomato sauce or mushroom sauce or spinach, steamed tomatoes, or Peperonata recipe.

Sauté onion in melted fat. Wash and sauté millet briefly with onion. Add water and cook over low heat for 20 min. Remove from stove and let swell for 10 min. Sprinkle cheese over millet or sauté onion strips until golden brown, and pour over all when ready to serve.

154. Millet Risotto with Vegetables (4 portions)

As in recipe 156, but with 1 cup diced vegetables (carrots, celery, leek, peas)
2 tbsp. cheese
1/2 oz. butter
1/2 onion, cut into rings

Sauté diced vegetables with onion and millet and cook until soft. Supplements in recipe No. 156.

155. Millet Pudding (4 portions)

7 oz. washed millet
1 qt. boiling milk
1 pinch sea salt
2 oz. butter
1-1/2-2 oz. fruit concentrate
3 egg yolks
1 tbsp. raisins
Some grated lemon peel (organically grown only)
3 beaten egg whites
1/2 oz. fresh butter
Compote

Add millet and salt to the boiling milk and cook over low heat. As soon as the milk is absorbed, remove from fire and let soak in completely while covered, for a total of 20 minutes. Cool in a bowl, but do not allow to become completely cold. Stir butter until frothy. Add in succession, fruit concentrate, egg yolks, raisins, lemon peel, mixing with the millet. Fold in egg whites carefully. Fill into buttered mold and place in a well preheated oven. Bake 40-60 min. at medium heat until uniformly golden brown. Dot top with butter. Serve with compote as a supplement.

156. Millet Dumplings (by Dr. Dorschner)
(4 portions)

2 cups millet (about 14 oz.)
4 cups water
2 minced onions
Mixed vegetables (carrots, celery root, leek, kohlrabi, white cabbage, etc.)
Garlic, herb or celery salt, marjoram, and a little cold-pressed sunflower seed oil

Cook millet in pressure cooker, together with onions, for about 30 minutes. Prepare vegetables while millet is cooking; stew, and mix with the soft cooked millet mash. Season with salt, marjoram and oil. Form dumplings with a small scoop and garnish with finely chopped parsley.

Millet is available at health food stores. 1 lb. is sufficient for 6 persons.

157. Polenta (4 portions)

7 oz. coarse cornmeal
1 qt. milk whey, or water and milk
1/2 tsp. sea salt
1 tbsp. fresh butter or margarine
1-2 tbsp. Swiss cheese or
Parmesan, or
1/2 oz. butter
1/2 onion, cut into rings

Mix cornmeal with cold whey and cook, covered, over low heat for 20 minutes. Remove from heat and let stand covered for 10 minutes. Mix in butter before serving. Grate cheese and sprinkle over polenta, or sauté onion until golden brown and lay on top of the polenta.

158. Cut Corn, Gratiné (4 portions)

Mixture mentioned above
1 oz. butter or diet margarine
2 tbsp. grated cheese
8-16 tbsp. coffee cream
Tomato sauce or tomatoes and salad

While hot, roll out on moist wooden board, 1/2 inch thick, let cool, cut into squares and lay like bricks in a flat, buttered, heat-resistant dish. Place butter patties on top. Sprinkle cheese over squares and pour coffee cream on top. Bake at a high temperature until a bright brown crust has formed. As a supplement, serve with tomatoes.

159. Fresh Corn on the Cob (4 portions)

Use only ears of corn whose kernels are tender and juicy.

4 ears of corn
1 qt. boiling water
1/2 tsp. sea salt
1 oz. fresh butter

Remove husk and silk from corn. Boil 20 min. or longer until corn is tender. Serve on a hot plate with fresh butter.

160. Whole Brown Semolina Gnocchi (3-4 portions)

Brown Semolina is rather dark and significantly more valuable than white semolina. It tastes very good and can certainly be used instead of white semolina. Available in health food stores.

6 oz. brown semolina
1/2 qt. milk
1/2 qt. water
1/2 tsp. sea salt
2 eggs (if allowed)
1/5 qt. milk or coffee cream
1 pinch sea salt
1 tbsp. grated cheese
1 oz. butter patties

Boil milk and water. Stir semolina into boiling liquid and cook 15-20 minutes. On a moistened board, roll out until about 1/2-3/4 in. thick, let cool, cut into squares or strips or carve round discs. Place the odd pieces in a buttered flat heat-resistant dish and then place the round discs over them. Beat milk and eggs together and pour over pieces. Sprinkle cheese over all. Place butter on top and bake at medium heat for about 20 min. until a golden-brown crust has formed.

161. Whole-Wheat Bread (to be baked at home)

When no whole-wheat bread can be obtained at the bakery, or its quality is unsatisfactory, excellent whole-wheat bread can be baked at home, whether the oven be gas, wood, or electric. The following instructions have been fully tested and proven. Naturally, more work is involved than if the bread were bought at the bakery, but you can also be more certain that it is prepared from completely fresh whole-wheat meal and contains its full natural value.

It is best to use organically grown grains. Keep the granules and remove the hard hulls, stones, or wooden parts, if they are found in the grain.

To make a loaf of about 3 pounds, take 2 pounds ground whole meal, 1/2 oz. pressed yeast, and a level tablespoon of salt; add a good half-quart of water. It is better to begin with this small amount until experience in kneading is acquired. Afterwards, two or more loaves can be baked at one time.

Grind the grain in a small house grain mill or coarse coffee mill or have it ground at a health food store. So that the whole-wheat bread does not become lumpy, but attains good consistency and can be cut easily, add a tablespoon of oil. This also gives the bread a pleasant taste.

Place the ground grain in a bowl, make a hole in the center, add the yeast, diluted with lukewarm water, (it must flow easily from the spoon), and mix it with some flour into a dough that is not too thick. Then add some more flour, so that a crust forms as it rises. Cover the bowl and place in a warm spot until the dough has taken well. Depending on the amount of heat, this takes 1-3 hours. Dissolve the salt in 1/2 quart lukewarm water and add the oil. Work the water into the meal slowly. When all the water is absorbed, knead the dough thoroughly for 15-20 minutes, constantly turning and twisting it until it is supple, yet firm. Finally, pound it on the table forcefully, about 20 times, lifting it up with both arms and pounding it on the table. Then put the dough back into the bowl and leave it in a warm place for another half-hour, forming a long loaf, and then place it in the greased or buttered cake pan which has also been dusted with flour (press down well). Leave it for 10-15 minutes. Fill the mold only 2/3 full, as the bread will rise. Bake at low heat in an oven that has been slightly preheated. The correct baking time varies with almost every oven and must be tested. The correct setting will be found if it takes about 2 hours for the bread to be ready. A shorter amount of time will create a hard crust and an unbaked inside; a longer time will dry the bread out.

Do not eat before the second day. It is good for 8 days, if stored in an airy, cool (not cold) spot.

In the same way, solid little loaves can also be baked: 1/2 qt. water and 1/2 qt. milk, instead of water and oil; also with 1 oz. butter. Form round spheres (about 3 oz. dough) and press flat. Baking time, 20-30 minutes.

Bread Spreads

162. Herb Butter (by Dr. Dorshner) (4 portions)

4-1/2 oz. health-food-store margarine
1 minced onion
Marjoram
Herb salt
Tomato pulp
Plenty of fresh minced herbs (such as parsley, chives, tarragon, pimpinella)

Beat margarine until frothy. Add onion to margarine. Mix all ingredients together well, and spread on slices of whole wheat bread.

163. Cream Cheese Spread (by Dr. Dorschner) (4 portions)

4-1/2 oz. health-food-store margarine
1 cream cheese, small
1 minced onion
Paprika, powdered
Seasoned salt

Mix well margarine, cheese, and onion. Season with paprika and salt.

164. Horseradish Butter (by Dr. Dorschner) (2 portions)

4 oz. health-food-store margarine
1 tbsp. finely grated horseradish

Mix all ingredients.
For cottage cheese spreads, see page 93.

Rice Dishes

We make the following distinctions:

1. Whole rice with an external, hard seed hull—spelt— is a very valuable food for stimulating the intestine, but suitable only for people accustomed to chewing well and who allow themselves time for calm eating.

Whole rice requires a very long time for soaking or cooking and therefore must not be sautéed beforehand in fat, otherwise it will no longer be soft. Cook with sautéed onions, in 2-1/2—3 times as much water as rice, and some sea salt. Pour the water cold over the rice, cook for 40 minutes. It then tastes excellent, hearty, and seasoned.

2. Whole rice without the external spelt, but with a valuable small silver hull and with full complement of vitamins and minerals is available as brown rice. It is well suited for risotto, rice fillings, rice soups, and other rice dishes and quickly turns soft. This whole rice is always referred to in the following recipes.

3. Vitaminized types of rice, such as Uncle Ben's Rice, among others, are completely hulled, but remain grainy and turn white on cooking.

4. A particular specialty of the highest value, a native American Indian food, is wild rice from natural soil, as the original Indians used to gather it, with long dark seeds. As a popular food, it cannot be considered today because of its high price, but as a special supplier of energy, it can still be recommended instead of a Sunday roast which is far more expensive.

165. Rice Salad (4 portions)

7 oz. whole rice
1 qt. boiling water
1 pinch sea salt
3 tbsp. oil
1-1/2 tbsp. lemon juice or
Health-food-store apple vinegar
1/2 tbsp. minced onion
1 pinch sea salt
2 tomatoes
Diced bell pepper
1 tsp. capers, if desired
Chives, basil
Large, healthy lettuce leaves

Wash rice very well, until water runs clear, before putting in boiling water. Add salt and do not cook it too soft. Put it in a sieve to rinse, and let it cool. Beat oil, lemon juice, onion, salt into a sauce, and mix with the rice. Dip the tomatoes into boiling water, peel, and dice fine. Dice pepper. Mix capers, chives and basil and mix everything gently with the rice. Season to taste. Serve the prepared rice salad on green lettuce leaves, perhaps garnished with tomato slices.

166. Rice Pudding (4 portions)

4 oz. rice
1/2 qt. boiling water
1/2 tsp. sea salt
1/4 qt. boiling milk
2 oz. butter or diet margarine
2 oz. fruit concentrate
Grated lemon peel
2 egg yolks
Possibly 1 tbsp. raisins
2 stiffly beaten egg whites
1/2 oz. butter

Wash rice well until water runs clear. Cook in boiling water and salt until half-soft. Pour water over rice to rinse, and finish cooking with boiling milk. The rice should still be somewhat grainy. Let cool. Beat, until frothy, butter, fruit concentrate, egg yolks, mix in the lemon peel and raisins, and mix with the rice before it is completely cold. Fold in the egg whites carefully last. Fill buttered pudding mold with rice mixture. Place butter patties on top and bake for 3/4 hr. at medium heat. As supplement, serve with compote.

167. Rice Pudding with Fruit (4 portions)

Mix the rice as above.
2 tart apples, cut into fine slices or fresh cherries or soaked dried apricots
1/2 oz. fresh butter

Fill a buttered pudding mold with the rice (as above) in alternating layers with the fruit and bake. Place butter patties on top.

168. Japanese Rice (4 portions)

9 oz. whole rice
5-6 cups water
1 pinch salt
1-1/2 oz. vegetable fat (if permitted)

Place rice in boiling water with salt and cook for 40 min. The rice should be grainy. Let cool; reheat on a cookie sheet in the oven. Dot with fat on top when ready to serve.

169. Rice Creole (4 portions)

9 oz. rice
5-6 cups water or vegetable broth
1 pinch salt

Place rice in boiling water or vegetable broth and cook until done.

170. Rice Creole with Vegetables (4 portions)

2 cups vegetables (celery root, leeks, and carrots), very finely diced
9 oz. rice
5-6 cups vegetable broth
1 pinch salt

Place everything in boiling vegetable broth and cook until done.

171. Tomato Rice (4 portions)

2 small tomatoes
1-1/4 cups rice
1 pinch salt
5 cups vegetable broth

Peel and dice tomatoes, and add to rice with salt. Add broth and cook.

172. Rice with Zucchini (4 portions)

1 lb. tender zucchini
Vegetable fat
3/4 cup vegetable broth or water
9 oz. rice

Dice zucchini and sauté briefly. Add rice, and gradually add more liquid as needed, until a risotto forms.

173. Rice with Spinach (4 portions)

1 tbsp. vegetable fat
14 oz. spinach (coarsely cut)
9 oz. rice
7 cups water or vegetable broth (hot)

Sauté spinach and rice. Add broth and cook.

174. Risotto (4 portions)

1-1/4 cups whole rice
2 tbsp. vegetable fat
1 chopped onion
5-6 cups vegetable broth or water
1 pinch sea salt
Rosemary
2 tbsp. grated cheese
Sweet butter, if desired

Wash rice thoroughly until water runs clear (3 times), and sauté with the onions until it is transparent. Add boiling broth, salt, and rosemary, and cook covered for 18 min. over low heat. Stir cheese through the rice with a fork before serving.

175. Risi-Bisi: Vegetable Rice (4 portions)

2 tbsp. vegetable fat
1 cup finely diced vegetables
   (celery root, leek, tomatoes, carrots, possibly mushrooms)
3/5 qt. vegetable broth
7 oz. whole rice
1 pinch sea salt

Sauté all vegetables together in fat. Add rice, salt, and boiling broth, and cook covered for 18 min. over low heat.

Warm and Cold Sauces

176. Herb Sauce (for 4 portions)

1 tbsp. butter
2 tbsp. whole meal
1 tbsp. white flour
2 cups vegetable bouillon or water
1 pinch sea salt
Yeast extract
2 tbsp. cream (if desired)

Melt butter. Stir in flour and sauté together. Add liquid slowly, and constantly stirring. Add salt, Cook 20 min. Stir in cream before serving.

177. Tomato Sauce (for 4 portions)

1 tbsp. vegetable fat
1 chopped onion
1-1/4 lb. ripe tomatoes
Some rosemary, thyme, basil, or 1 sage leaf
1 pinch sea salt
1 pinch sugar
1 tsp. cornstarch
2 tbsp. cream (if desired)

Melt fat and sauté onions in it. Cut tomatoes into slices, sauté together until soft. Strain and add herbs, salt and sugar. Stir in cornstarch and cook for a few minutes. Stir in cream before serving.

178. Tomato Sauce II (4 portions)

18 oz. ripe tomatoes
1 pinch sea salt
Some rosemary, thyme, basil, or 1 sage leaf
1 pinch sugar
2 tbsp. cream (if desired)

Cut into pieces. cook with herbs, salt and sugar until soft; strain. Stir in cream before serving.

179. Raw Tomato Sauce (4 portions)

18 oz. ripe tomatoes (especially suitable, are Italian plum tomatoes)
1 tsp. lemon juice
1 pressed clove of garlic
1 pinch sea salt
1 pinch sugar
A little rosemary, thyme, chives, basil, or 1 sage leaf
Grated horseradish, if desired

Strain tomatoes or blend in electric blender. Mix with the other ingredients. Add herbs, depending on choice, minced. Do not cook this sauce, but you may warm it gently if desired.

Sweet Dishes
(Without Refined Sugar)

Whenever possible, use concentrated pear juice, fruit concentrate, honey, or dried fruit for sweetening instead of sugar. Usually, it takes only a short amount of time to become accustomed to this, so that the longing for excessive sweetening disappears. Healthy instincts will soon lean toward the less-sweetened dishes rather than excessively sweetened ones.

A mere one hundred years ago, it was not customary to use a lot of sugar. We gather this from a report on diet in the Zurich highlands: "The farmers' wives cooked all fruit without adding sugar: apples, plums, cherries, and elderberries. A large ladle of whole dark flour was mixed with milk and added to the cooking compote, in order to tone down the taste of the fruit acids."

Fruits

180. Fruit Compote (from an old recipe without sugar)
(4 portions)

2 lbs. fruit (blueberries, cherries, tart apples, rhubarb)
1/2 cup water
1-2 tbsp. whole wheat flour
1 cup whole milk
Some honey or pear juice
1 oz. butter
Bread cubes
Cream

Bring fruit to boil in water. Blend flour with the milk into a smooth paste and add to the fruit. Bring to a boil once more. Let cool. Sweeten to taste with honey or pear juice. Melt butter and sauté bread cubes in it. Scatter cubes over the cooled fruit compote. Serve cream with fruit to tone down the taste of the fruit acids.

181. Blueberry or Cherry Dish (4 portions)

2 lbs. fruit
Water
1 tbsp. butter
2 tbsp. whole wheat flour
Concentrated pear juice
1/2 oz. butter
1/2 oz. bread cubes

Boil fruit in water and set fruit aside. Blend flour and butter, sauté together, and mix with the juice of the boiled fruit. Bring to boil again and add fruit. Sweeten to taste. Sauté bread cubes in butter and scatter over the dish. Serve warm.

This dish can also be prepared with plums, apricots, and tart, stewed apples. The taste of the dish can be improved by adding ground almonds cooked with the other ingredients and by adding some finely grated lemon peel.

182. Fruit Salad (4 portions)

2-4 tbsp. concentrated pear-juice or fruit-juice concentrate,
Or 1/2-1 cup date juice
1 cup water and 1 cup grape juice
1 tbsp. lemon juice
1-3/4 lbs. apricots, peaches, prunes, plums, oranges
Or, tangerines, apples, melons, bananas
2 tbsp. raisins
2 tbsp. pine kernels or sunflower seeds

Bring sweetener to a boil with the water, let cool; add some grape juice if desired. Mixed or single fruit, cut in halves, slices, or cubes. Slice apples thinly, place in the cool syrup, and let them soak. Add raisins and nuts according to taste.

183. Cold Fruit Soup (raw compote) (4 portions)

1-3/4 lbs. soft fruit: peaches, apricots, bananas, oranges, berries
1 cup apple or grape juice
1 tbsp. lemon juice
4 tbsp. almond cream or cream
2-3 tbsp. pear-juice or fruit-juice concentrate, or 8 tbsp. date juice

Use only one kind of fruit; do not mix. Press one half of the fruit through a sieve or mash. Mix juice with the fruit pulp. Add lemon juice if desired. Add cream. Sweeten to taste with juice concentrate. Cut the remaining half of the fruit into slices or cubes, but leave berries whole, and place in the raw fruit sauce.

184. Creamed Bananas (4 portions)

About 1 qt. yogurt, or coffee cream, or almond cream
2-3 tbsp. lemon juice
1 tsp. honey, if desired
8 ripe bananas

Mix together yogurt, honey, and lemon juice. Beat 4 bananas until frothy, with a fork. Cut the other 4 into discs and arrange in layers.

185. Junket with Fruit (4 portions)

1 qt. milk
1-2 tbsp. raw sugar
Vanilla sugar or grated lemon peel
1 junket tablet
1 cup fresh berries
8 tbsp. cream

Warm milk and flavoring to about 98.6 degrees F. Crush junket tablet, dissolve in water and place in the warm milk; pour immediately into glasses. When junket is set, refrigerate. Garnish with berries and cream.

186. Banana and Apple Creme with Cottage Cheese
(4 portions)

4 oz. cream or skim cottage cheese
Milk or yogurt, if needed
4 bananas
4 sour juicy apples
Grated lemon peel, cinnamon, or ginger as desired
1 tsp. honey, if desired

Blend cheese and yogurt or milk until smooth. Beat bananas with a fork until frothy. Grate apples very fine. Mix all ingredients well, or blend in a blender.

For fruit cream with cottage cheese, see recipe 71.

187. Stuffed Baked Apples (4 portions)

4 large or 8 small apples
4 tbsp. crushed hazelnuts
2 tbsp. raisins
4 tbsp. coffee cream or yogurt
2 tbsp. pear juice
Grated lemon peel
1/2 oz. butter patties
1 tbsp. pear juice
8-16 tbsp. apple juice

Mix nuts, raisins, cream or yogurt, lemon peel, and stuff into apples. Place in a heat resistant flat dish. Distribute pear juice and butter patties over apples. Fill dish with sweet cider to about 1/2 in. high and bake for 20-30 min.

188. Red Grits (for 4 portions)

6 cups currant, raspberry, or strawberry juice,
    or a mixture of them
1/2 cup red grape juice
3 tbsp. pear juice
2-1/2 oz. semolina
1 tbsp. cornstarch
Certified milk, coffee cream, or almond milk.

Boil all juices together. Mix semolina and cornstarch together dry. Add to boiling juice while stirring. Boil 10 min. Pour into a rinsed pudding mold and let cool until firm. Unmold. Add milk or cream as supplement if desired.

189. Cherry Pudding (4 portions)

7 oz. whole wheat bread
2-3 tbsp. milk
4 oz. butter or diet margarine
4 oz. pear juice concentrate
3-4 egg yolks
9 oz. cherries
2 oz. grated almonds
1 tsp. cinnamon
1 tbsp. cherry juice
3-4 egg whites

Crumble bread, moisten with milk, and put through a blender. Beat margarine, juice concentrate, egg yolks, until frothy, stir in little by little. Mix all ingredients well. Beat egg whites until stiff and fold carefully into the mixture. Fill buttered pudding mold and bake for 40 min. in the oven at medium heat.

190. Dutch Currant Bread (4 portions)

14 oz. strained whole wheat flour
3 oz. butter or diet margarine
1 pinch sea salt
1 tbsp. raw sugar
3/4 oz. yeast
2 cups lukewarm milk
7 oz. currants
5 oz. raisins
3 tbsp. flour
2 oz. diced candied lemon peel
1-1/4 cups milk
2 eggs

Place flour, salt, and sugar in a warm bowl. Make a depression in the center. Divide butter into small pieces on the flour. Dissolve yeast and put it in the center of the flour. Make a thin dough with some flour, milk, and yeast, and set in a warm place, covered, until the dough has doubled in size. Wash currants and dust with the flour. Mix currants and raisins, lemon peel, milk, and eggs with the dough. Fill a greased cake pan with the mixture; let it rise once again, and bake for about 1 hr.

Cut into slices when cold and serve with or without butter or, if desired, also with honey at breakfast or dinner.

191. Millet Pudding with Fruit (4 portions)

Dough of millet pudding (see recipe 164)
2-4 sour apples, peeled or 2 cups presoaked dried apricots
Some raw sugar to taste

Fill a well-buttered pudding mold in alternate layers with finely sliced apples or precooked dried apricots and some raw sugar. Bake as directed above.

10 butter patties—Use as above.
Apple Rice Pudding—See recipe 167.
Cottage Cheese Pudding—See recipe 73.
Cottage Cheese Cake—See recipe 195.

Cakes and Tortes

192. Nut and Fruit Torte (4 portions)

Pitted dates or figs or raisins or apricots, or a mixture
Hazelnuts or almonds

Crush and press nuts through a grinder. A kneadable dough should form. Roll out, cover bottom of pie dish, and let cool. Before eating, top with fresh fruit. Place a bit of agar-agar over this. Finally, garnish with some whipped cream.

193. Carrot Torte (by Dr. Dorschner) (4 portions)

9 oz. grated carrots
9 oz. grated hazelnuts
5 egg yolks
5 oz. honey
1/2 tsp. cinnamon
1 pinch salt
5 egg whites

Mix all ingredients well except egg whites. Beat egg whites medium stiff into a light snow, fold into mixture, bake for about 45 min. at a medium heat.

194. Hazelnut Ring (by Dr. Dorschner) (4 portions)

11 oz. whole wheat flour
2 level tsp. baking powder
3 oz. honey
1 egg
2 tbsp. milk or water
4-1/2 oz. margarine
Filling:
    7 oz. ground hazelnuts
    3 oz. honey
    4-5 drops baking oil
    Bitter almonds
1 egg yolk

Make a kneaded dough from the ingredients and roll out into a rectangle of about 14 by 18 in. Mix nuts, honey, oil, and almonds with enough water to form a pliant dough. With a plastic spoon, dipping it into water frequently, spread the mixture out on the unrolled dough. Roll up the dough from the longer side, fashion into a ring on a greased baking sheet and brush with a beaten egg yolk. Baking Time: 40-45 min. at a good medium heat.

195. Cottage Cheese Cake (4 portions)

9 oz. butter or sugar dough or grated dough as described
3/4 oz. butter
2-1/2 oz. fruit concentrate
3-4 oz. almonds
18 oz. cottage cheese
2 egg yolks
2 tbsp. cornstarch
2 oz. raisins
1 pinch sea salt
Possibly some vanilla sugar
2 beaten egg whites

Roll out and lay dough in a cake pan. Beat butter until frothy with fruit concentrate. Peel and grate almonds. Mix all ingredients well, except egg whites. Fold in egg whites last. Place the cottage cheese mass on the dough and bake for 3/4 hr. at low heat.

Sweet Sauces

196. Almond Milk Sauce (4 portions)

2 cups milk
2 oz. shelled, grated almonds
1-1/2 oz. fruit concentrate
1 tbsp. cornstarch
2 tbsp. water

Boil milk. Add almonds and boil with milk. Mix cornstarch with water and then stir into the boiling milk. Mix with the prepared sauce, so that it becomes creamy, soft, and frothy.

197. Rose Hip Sauce (4 portions)

2-1/2 oz. rose hip pulp, unsweetened
Pear juice to taste
1-3/4 cups water or grape juice
A few drops of lemon juice

Bring all to a boil together. Drip lemon juice into the prepared sauce.

198. Apricot Sauce (for 4 portions)

9 oz. apricot compote
Pear juice (instead of sugar) for sweetening to taste
1-2 tbsp. cream

Strain through a sieve or blend in a blender, dilute with the juice. Add to soften the taste of the acids.

199. Fruit Sauce (for 4 portions)

Fruit juice concentrate
Grape or apple juice
Pear juice concentrate
1 tbsp. cornstarch
2 tbsp. water

Dilute with the grape or apple juice to taste, bring to a boil. For sweetening. Blend cornstarch with water, add slowly to the boiling fruit sauce, bring to a boil, let cool.

Beverages

Health Teas

200. Bitter Tea

Wormwood
Centaury
Common Benedict (Blessed Thistle)

Mix teas in equal parts, boil and let stand for 5 minutes. In case of loss of appetite, drink 2-3 tbsp., 1/2 hr. before meals. Slightly choleretic and therefore therapeutic for migraines.

201. Gas-Relieving Tea

Caraway seed
Fennel
Anise

Mix in equal parts. Pour boiling water over seeds, and let steep for 20 min. Drink 1 cup after meals.

202. Camomile Tea

Pour boiling water over dried flowerets. Steep only. Use for abdominal pains. Purifying and calming to the gastrointestinal tract. Good for enemas and affusions externally.

203. Peppermint Tea

Steep only. Calming and choleretic. Popular pleasant tea.

204. Verbena Tea

Steep only. Calming, phlegm reducing, choleretic. Very popular pleasant tea in France.

205. Solidago (Golden Rod) Tea

Boil 1 min., let steep 10 min. For dropsy, kidney, and bladder infections. Diuretic, 2-3 cups daily.

206. Rose Hip Tea

Soak 2-3 tbsp. rose hip seeds and shells in 1-1/2 qts. water for 12 hrs., then gently boil for 1/2-3/4 hr. Strain. The rest of the cooked rose hips can advantageously be boiled again with fresh rose hips on the following day. Slightly choleretic and diuretic. Very suitable with meals because of its slightly tart flavor.

207. Blueberry Tea

Dried berries

Soak 12 hrs., boil 10 min. in water, steep 15-30 min. Disinfecting, stops diarrhea and calming to the intestine.

208. Linseed Tea

1 tbsp. to 1/2 qt. water. Boil 7-10 min. and steam for a short time. Reduces phlegm, slightly laxative. In the case of stomach infections and rather long juice fasts, add raw fruit juices to 1/3 linseed puree. Tones down the taste of the fruit acids.

Sedative Teas

209. Lemon Peel Tea

Peel of one lemon for 2 cups tea. Wash unsprayed lemons and grate well, then peel thinly like potato peelings. Steep in boiling water and set aside for 5 min., then strain. Drink with some honey before going to sleep.

210. Golden Sassafrass Tea

Steep only and set aside for 5 min. Drink with some honey before going to sleep.

211. Orange Blossom Tea

Boil 2-3 blossoms 2-3 min., steep a short time and strain. Sweeten with honey and drink before going to sleep.

Additional recipes can be found in the other Bircher-Benner Handbooks.

V. Exercises

In all head exercises, the cervical vertebrae should be straight. The shoulders should be horizontal and back. Do the exercises very slowly.

In exercises 1, 2, and 3, concentrate on the weight of the head. This draws the head lower and lower and stretches neck muscles to a maximum. Without causing cramps, stop in a stretched position for a few seconds, at first—later for 1-2 minutes. The idea that strongly stretched muscle fibers are like rubber bands that give more and more, can be of help.

1) Let the head fall forward.
2) Let the head fall backward.
3) Let the head fall sideways, while keeping your face pointing forward. (Use a mirror for control.)
4) Turn the head slowly as far as possible to left and right while keeping cervical vertebrae straight. The collarbone should remain still.

This exercise achieves new body posture especially in the neck area. Sit against a wall, with back, rib cage, and the back of the head in contact with the wall. Place the feet slightly forward.

1) Press feet down with the whole soles slanting into the floor. In this way, the cervical vertebrae are slowly directed upward. They are also stretched by this pressure. No force is needed except for the slight pressure of the feet on the floor.
2) Letting up on the pressure of the feet, round the shoulders slightly and roll the head back to an apex, lifting the chin.

Alternate exercises 1) and 2) several times in slow rhythm.

Other Nash Quality Paperbacks Related to Health and Nutrition You'll Be Sure to Enjoy

THE MAGIC OF HONEY by Dorothy Perlman. The ancients appreciated the glorious taste of honey — symbol of love in story, music and poetry. Health-food enthusiasts have discovered, once again, honey's powers — its delicious flavor, medicinal qualities and natural nutritional values. Here is everything you'd like to know about honey: it's role in history, its wondrous energy- and health-giving attributes, its legendary possibilities as a fertility food and aphrodisiac.   #8001 $1.95

ORGANIC MAKE-UP by Mary Gjerde. Whatever your age or skin type, nature provides an aid to protect and enhance your skin. Honey, eggs and milk; plant substances such as herbs, fruits, leaves and seeds; extracts and rich oils of almond, avocado and olive are all natural materials intended by nature for you to use on your skin and hair. And you will find all of these natural ingredients in your own kitchen at a fraction of the cost charged for their synthetic counterparts.   #8003 $1.95

VITAMIN E: KEY TO SEXUAL SATISFACTION by Gary P. Brandner. Everyone's talking about Vitamin E. Here is a revealing account of how and why the amazing "E" has come to be known as "the sex vitamin." If a vitamin can be called topical, Vitamin E is just that. The author traces its history and documents how it heightens sexual capabilities and increases response and sensitivity during sexual encounters.   #8000 $1.95

INTRODUCTION TO HEALTH FOODS by Marjorie Miller. This complete guide on how to prepare and enjoy health foods introduces the novice to the various types and forms of health foods, their nutritional value, the dangers of artificial preservatives, general principles of good nutrition, how to cook food so it doesn't lose its value, and exactly what foods are found in a health food store.   #1187 $2.45

INTRODUCTION TO ORGANIC GARDENING by Chuck Pendergast. The author shows how organic gardening will improve the quality of the foods we eat and help restore the natural balance which has been destroyed by the use of pesticides and chemical fertilizers. Illustrates how to grow your own fruit and vegetables the safe, healthy and natural way.   #1188 $2.45

Now at your bookstore or order from Nash Publishing, 9255 Sunset Boulevard, Los Angeles, California 90069. Add 40c per book for shipping.

Announcing
a New Solution to the Common Cold by Dale Alexander:

The Common Cold and Common Sense

Vitamin C is only part of the answer, claims Dale Alexander in this revolutionary work dealing with the common cold. Author of the best seller, Arthritis and Common Sense, Dale Alexander presents a totally new understanding of the common cold, including nutritional secrets that he contends will not only help prevent your catching cold but will ensure your general good health.

If you follow Dale Alexander's sensible, pleasant, nutritional regimen and pay heed to what he claims causes the common cold, the author maintains that the results will be greatly desired good health — free of colds — and the ability to function on all fronts. #1172 $5.95

Now at your bookstore or order from Nash Publishing, 9255 Sunset Boulevard, Los Angeles, California 90069. Add 40c per book for shipping.

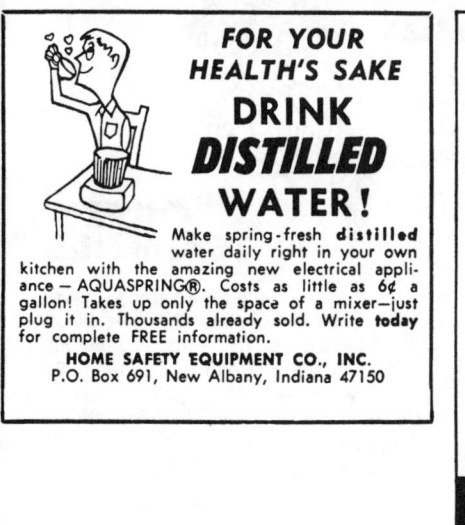

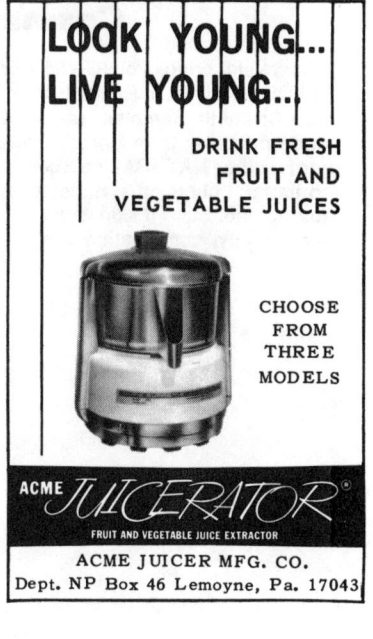

FOR YOUR HEALTH'S SAKE DRINK *DISTILLED* WATER!

Make spring-fresh **distilled** water daily right in your own kitchen with the amazing new electrical appliance — AQUASPRING®. Costs as little as 6¢ a gallon! Takes up only the space of a mixer—just plug it in. Thousands already sold. Write **today** for complete FREE information.

HOME SAFETY EQUIPMENT CO., INC.
P.O. Box 691, New Albany, Indiana 47150

LOOK YOUNG... LIVE YOUNG...

DRINK FRESH FRUIT AND VEGETABLE JUICES

CHOOSE FROM THREE MODELS

ACME *JUICERATOR*®
FRUIT AND VEGETABLE JUICE EXTRACTOR

ACME JUICER MFG. CO.
Dept. NP Box 46 Lemoyne, Pa. 17043

Randall Back To Nature

HYPO-ALLERGENIC NUTRITIONAL COSMETICS SINCE 1950

"Doggone Good"

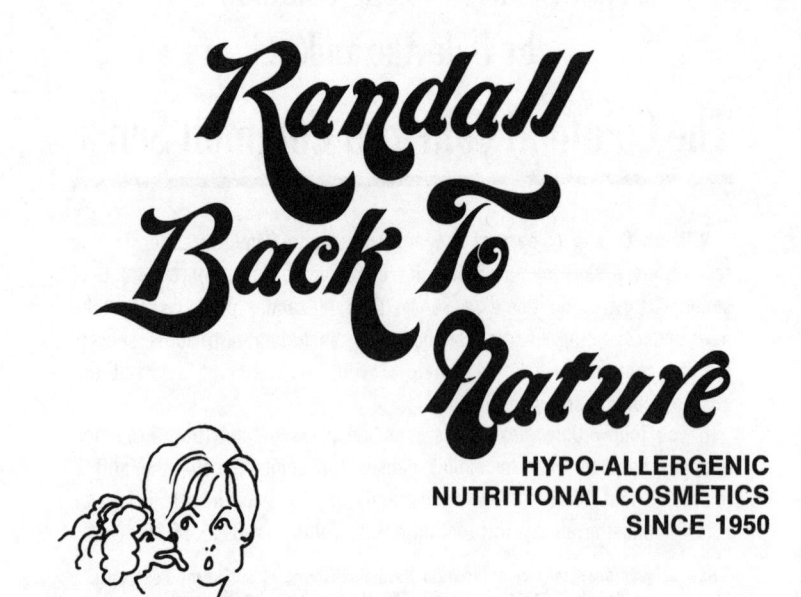

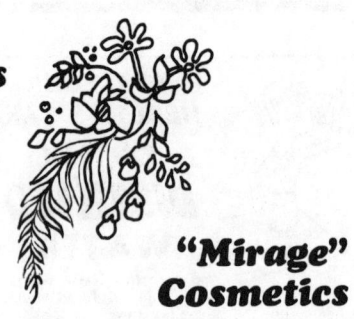

Randall Cosmetics

Only $1 still brings you 9 - 25¢ TRY-BEFORE-YOU-BUY Randall basic skin care Cosmetic Samples (save $1.25). Made primarily from Herbs, Flowers, Ferns, other NATURAL sources; no harmful chemicals. Satisfaction guaranteed. State if skin is dry, normal, oily, combination.

"Mirage" Cosmetics

Send only $6 for the $1 set of 9 Randall Cosmetic Samples PLUS the $9 size (2-drams) of fabulous "Mirage" Beauty Lotion ($11.25 value—save $5.25). Mrs. A. S. of Charlotte, N.C., writes: "Mirage should be called "Miracle"—it does wonders!" Prepaid. Satisfaction guaranteed.

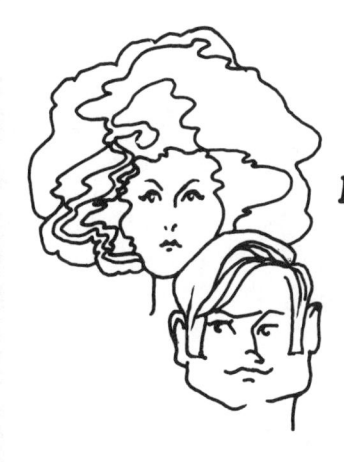

Eighteen Natural-Organic Creme Hair Colors

Natural-Organic Hair Permanents

At long last, Natural-Organic Hair Colors free from analine and metallic dyes; Permanents with no thiaglycolic acid nor its salts. N.G. of Portland, Ore. writes: "Your color treatment is fantastic. This is the first time in years my scalp hasn't been burning, itching, scaling, etc., after coloring—and to think, this condition cleared up with only one application. I am delighted." Write for complete FREE information. No obligation, of course.

CHECK YOUR LOCAL HEALTH STORE
OR ORDER FROM

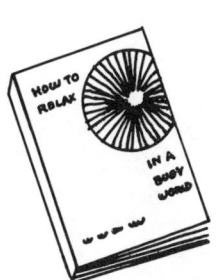

Randall Back To Nature

7924 IVANHOE AVENUE
LA JOLLA, CALIFORNIA 92037
PHONE: (714) 454-4003

"HOW TO RELAX IN A BUSY WORLD"

Dr. Floyd Corbin, noted blind Philosopher, Humorist, Lecturer, and his many-talented wife, Eve, are both listed in "WHO'S WHO in California." Their message: "Everything can be better for you"—and they show you HOW! New edition, only $3.00.